张耕铭 著

Written by
Zhang Gengming

中药免疫疗法癌前介入与核心技术单元支持概述
《伤寒论》对现代临床医学的启示

The Outline of
Precancerous
Intervention
and Core Technical
Unit Support
for TCM
Immunotherapy

The Enlightenment
of *Shanghan Lun*
to Modern Clinical Medicine

汉英双语版
Chinese-English Edition

全 国 百 佳 图 书 出 版 单 位
中国中医药出版社
·北京·

图书在版编目（CIP）数据

中药免疫疗法癌前介入与核心技术单元支持概述:《伤寒论》对现代临床医学的启示：汉、英 / 张耕铭著 . —北京：中国中医药出版社，2023.3
ISBN 978 – 7 – 5132 – 7988 – 8

Ⅰ . ①中… Ⅱ . ①张… Ⅲ . ①中药疗法—肿瘤免疫疗法 Ⅳ . ① R243 ② R730.51

中国版本图书馆 CIP 数据核字（2022）第 246555 号

中国中医药出版社出版
北京经济技术开发区科创十三街 31 号院二区 8 号楼
邮政编码　100176
传真　010-64405721
山东临沂新华印刷物流集团有限责任公司印刷
各地新华书店经销

开本 787×1092　1/32　印张 5.25　字数 90 千字
2023 年 3 月第 1 版　2023 年 3 月第 1 次印刷
书号　ISBN 978 – 7 – 5132 – 7988 – 8

定价　39.00 元
网址　www.cptcm.com

服 务 热 线　010-64405510
购 书 热 线　010-89535836
侵 权 打 假　010-64405753

微信服务号　zgzyycbs
微商城网址　https://kdt.im/LIdUGr
官 方 微 博　http://e.weibo.com/cptcm
天猫旗舰店网址　https://zgzyycbs.tmall.com
如有印装质量问题请与本社出版部联系（010-64405510）
版权专有　侵权必究

若夫法天则地,随应而动,和之者若响,随之者若影,道无鬼神,独来独往。

——《素问·宝命全形论》

If one can apply the therapy according to the principle of the variations of Yin and Yang of heaven and earth, the curative effects will be obtained as a matter of course. This is nothing mysterious, when one is serious in accumulating knowledges with protracted experience, something unique in his achievement will certainly occur.

— *Baoming Quanxing Lun of Suwen*

生生不息……

生命的起源和进化理论源远流长、众说纷纭，不过各种理论都可以归结为生生不息，生物总会找到办法繁衍生息。

我想请你们花点时间想想，对于肿瘤来说，我们也是麻烦，我们是入侵者，我们是它所面临的危险，对于肿瘤来说，我们才是癌症！

而肿瘤自己呢？肿瘤将自己视为一个努力想要来到这个世界的甜美的、可爱的、胖胖的婴儿，而我们想要阻止它、消灭它，像野蛮人一样把它从幸福温暖的小窝中撕取出来。

对于肿瘤来说，我们就是没有人性的、残忍的怪物。我为什么要这样说？我为什么叫它"婴儿"并在这里讨论如何"杀死"它？因为这种肿瘤值得我们尊重，值得被给予一点人性。

它不仅仅是个肿瘤，它足智多谋，它很强大，它有超凡的适应能力，它富有诗意，它是上帝的杰作，它是一个生命。和其他生命一样，它想生存，和其他生命一样，它会拼死求生……

——《实习医生格蕾》

Life will out...

The origins and lessons of life and evolution are long and complex, but what they basically boil down to is life will out, life will always find a way to continue.

I'd like you for one moment to consider the idea that, to the tumor, we are the problem, we are the invader, we are the danger, to the tumor, we are the cancer!

And the tumor? Well, the tumor sees itself as a sweet, cute, fat-cheeked baby, just trying to make its way into the world, and we want to stop it, destroy it, tear it from its happy little home like barbarians.

To the tumor, we are the soulless, murderous monsters. Why do I do this? Why do I call it a "baby" and talk about "killing" it? Because this kind of tumor deserves respect, it deserves a little humanity.

It's not just a tumor, it has ingenuity, strength, adaptability and poetry, it's one of god's masterpieces, it's alive. And like any living thing, it wants to stay alive, like any living thing, it is going to fight like hell to survive...

— *Grey's Anatomy*

内容简介

鉴于现代临床医学恶性肿瘤的高发率与高死亡率，作者通过对当前免疫疗法前沿思想与技术的分析，把握癌前病变的基本概念及最佳切入点，明晰癌症防治的核心突破点，讨论了现代医学筛查与诊断的空缺及诸多不足，深入发挥中医"治未病"与宏观诊断、调控方面的优势，并结合中医经典《伤寒论》与《黄帝内经》深度发掘中医瞑眩反应介入的临床机理与诊疗优势，依托六经辨证对癌前病变诊察、病因、病位、病机、治法加以探讨与归纳，从而总结出系统而又较为全面的中药免疫治疗方案，最终进一步论述了癌前病变的相关心理社会干预，形成了比较完备的临床医学思路，为"现代医学中医化"与"肿瘤防治六经化"做出了典范，为肿瘤免疫疗法提供了进一步开拓的可能性与颠覆性延伸，为人类生命健康发展提供切实可靠的保障。

Content Introduction

In view of the high incidence rate and high mortality of malignant tumors in modern clinical medicine, the author has grasped the basic concept and the best entry point of precancerous lesions, clarified the core breakthrough point of cancer prevention and treatment, discussed the gaps and many shortcomings of modern medical screening and diagnosis, and given full play to the advantages of "preventive treatment of disease", macroscopic diagnosis, and readjustment and control of TCM according to the analysis of the frontier ideas and techniques of immunotherapy. Referring to *Shanghan Lun* and *Huangdi Neijing*, the medical literatures from ancient China, the author has deeply explored clinical mechanism and advantages of intervention in dizziness reaction of TCM, and discussed and summarized the diagnosis, etiology, location, pathogenesis and treatment of precancerous lesions according to the six-meridian syndrome differentiation. Thus, a systematic and comprehensive immunotherapy scheme of TCM is summarized. Finally, the psycho-social intervention of precancerous lesions is further discussed, thus, a relatively complete clinical medical train of thought is formed, which makes a model for "modern medicine in a TCM way" and "tumor prevention and treatment in the six meridians way", provides the possibility of further development and subversive extension of tumor immunotherapy, and provides a practical and reliable guarantee for the health development of human life.

自序

中医最大的特色就是借自然顺势之为调整人体循环，尊重人体本身，达到与疾病背后非自然态势的和解。这就像是一条灵动的"生命线"，把复杂的病理反应串成了一条"项链"，保证了诊疗的"一贯性"，也为患者生命质量的提高提供了最大幅度的关怀与支持。

这部概述以癌前病变这一大病种为研究对象，以《伤寒论》理法方药为硬核思想，高度凝炼了中医六经辨证、卫气营血辨证、脏腑经络辨证的核心内涵，并充分结合了现代医学的辅助诊断与治疗，是笔者临证读书数载的智慧结晶，寒灯暗夜，一纸收尽，手册虽小，深藏玄机。

"真传一句话，假传万卷书""冗繁削尽留清瘦"，笔者秉着"临床方向多样化、临床操作简单化、临证思维极限化"的基本原则，提炼其最核心的临证思想，摒弃中医理论的繁杂化，力求以最精简、最系统的阐述方式还现代中医临床一个一清二白。

笔者对于从零开始积累纯中医治疗癌症经验的辛酸苦

Introduction

The biggest characteristic of TCM is to adjust the circulation of human body with the help of natural homeopathy to reconcile with the disease on the basis of respecting the human body itself. This is like a flexible "lifeline", which strings the complex pathological reactions into a "necklace", ensures the consistency of diagnosis and treatment, and also provides the greatest care and support for the improvement of the patients' life quality.

This outline takes the precancerous lesion as the research object, takes the theory, method, prescription and medicine of *Shanghan Lun* as the core thought, highly condenses the core content of the six-meridian syndrome differentiation, Wei-Qi-Ying-Blood syndrome differentiation, Zang-fu and meridians syndrome differentiation, and fully draws experience from the auxiliary diagnosis and treatment of modern medicine, which is the wisdom crystallization of the author's clinical and reading experience. Although the manual is small, it contains profound life mysteries, and countless dark nights of the author under the cold lamp are printed in it.

As the saying goes: "Wisdom is to make knowledge easy and clear; Stupidity is to make knowledge hard and intricate", "Truth is the core and essential thing left after all irrelevant

闷体会颇深，整个过程是非常惨痛的。如果每一个中医人都从零开始做起，对于患者而言将是巨大的代价。笔者衷心希望这套核心技术单元支持的整理总结能够为现代中医肿瘤临床的深入探索带来一些启发和帮助。

同时为了方便西学中及国外中医学习爱好者及临床人士参考学习，笔者利用空余时间特意将原文精心翻译为英文以双语对照形式刊出。另本概述处方中用药剂量与配伍形式为笔者针对特定疾病的独特经验，读者务必要辩证看待应用，切不可盲目照搬。

2022 年 12 月

interferences have been eliminated", the author holds on to the basic principles of "diversification of clinical direction, simplification of clinical operation, and maximization of clinical thinking", refines the core clinical thought, discards the complexity of TCM theory, and strives to make the modern TCM clear in the most concise and systematic way.

The author has deep experiences of accumulating experience in the treatment of cancer with traditional Chinese medicine from scratch, and the whole process could be said to be extremely painful. If every TCM clinician starts from scratch like the author, it will be a huge price for the patient. The author sincerely hopes that the outline can bring some inspiration and help to the further exploration of the clinical treatment of the tumor in the modern Chinese medicine.

In order to facilitate readers to refer to and quote, the author makes use of his spare time to translate the original text into English and publishes them in bilingual form. In addition, it should be noted that the dosage and compatibility of Chinese medicine in the decoction in this outline is the author's unique experience for specific diseases, the readers must treat and apply them dialectically and should not copy them blindly.

Zhang Gengming
Dec, 2022

目录

引言 — 001

一、癌前病变的相关基础概念 — 008

二、癌前病变现代临床筛查与诊断的空缺 — 012

三、"柳暗花明又一村"——中医瞑眩反应介入的临床机理与诊疗优势 — 016

四、中医辨证观下癌前阶段的常见特征性病理表现 — 038

五、中医辨证观下癌前病变病因的探讨 — 046

六、中医辨证观下癌前病变病位的探讨 — 050

七、中医辨证观下癌前病变病机的探讨 — 056

八、中医辨证观下癌前病变治法的探讨 — 072

九、中药免疫疗法癌前介入的基本原则与代表方剂 — 076

十、九鼎归宗饮加减与服药须知 — 080

十一、中药免疫疗法癌前介入的治疗转归 — 084

十二、中药免疫疗法癌前介入的瞑眩反应及其基本处理原则 — 094

十三、癌前病变的心理社会干预 — 138

十四、结语 — 146

参考文献 — 150

Catalogue

Preface	001
I. The Basic Concepts Related to Precancerous Lesions	009
II. The Defect of Modern Clinical Screening and Diagnosis of Precancerous Lesions	013
III. "There is a Way Out" — The Clinical Mechanism and the Diagnosis and Treatment Advantages of TCM in Dizziness Reaction Intervention	017
IV. Common Characteristic Pathological Manifestations of Precancerous Stage under the View of Syndrome Differentiation in TCM	039
V. Discussion on the Etiology of Precancerous Lesions under the View of Syndrome Differentiation in TCM	047
VI. Discussion on the Location of Precancerous Lesions under the View of Syndrome Differentiation in TCM	051
VII. Discussion on the Pathogenesis of Precancerous Lesions under the View of Syndrome Differentiation in TCM	057
VIII. Discussion on the Treatment of Precancerous Lesions under the View of Syndrome Differentiation in TCM	073
IX. The Basic Principles and Representative Formulas of Precancerous Intervention in Immunotherapy of TCM	077
X. Variations of Jiuding Guizong Decoction and Instructions for Taking Medicine	081
XI. Treatment Stages of Precancerous Intervention in Immunotherapy of TCM	085
XII. Dizziness Reactions and Their Basic Treatment Principles of Precancerous Intervention in Immunotherapy of TCM	095
XIII. Psycho-social Intervention of Precancerous Lesions	139
XIV. Conclusion	147

引言　　Preface

众所周知，在现代诸多慢性痼疾与疑难症中，恶性肿瘤已成为威胁人类健康和生命的主要疾病，多年来晚期癌症生存率总体来讲并无太大提高。我国主张抗癌战略前移，力争早期发现和早期治疗，癌前阶段正是其中的重要环节。因此，提升对癌症前期改变的认识，并对其做出准确诊断和及时有效的临床处理显得尤为重要。

伴随着现代肿瘤医学的多维度、综合性诊疗技术与手段的发展，中医学在肿瘤的临床治疗方面发挥着越来越为人所熟知与公认的不可替代的强大作用。继癌症免疫疗法荣获 2018 年诺贝尔生理学或医学奖后，免疫疗法也有望成为目前最有希望治愈癌症的精准化手段，但由于相关免疫药物在临床药理实验中的复杂性、多方向性与不可控性，致使免疫疗法依旧有许多亟待解决的问题，如 CAR-T、PD-1 等的复发可能性及毒性反应等导致的临床受众和远期疗效受限，同时免疫疗法的耐药性以及昂贵的成本也是不容忽视的问题。而随之带给中医药的创新机遇与独特优势则开始以未知的速度生根萌芽。

As we all know, in many modern chronic and difficult diseases, malignant tumors have become the main diseases threatening human health and life, and the survival rate of advanced cancer has not improved much over the years. Our country advocates implementing anticancer strategy ahead of time, strives for early detection and early treatment, and the precancerous stage is one of the important links. Therefore, it is particularly important to improve the understanding of precancerous changes, to make accurate diagnosis, and to take the timely and effective clinical treatment.

With the development of multi-dimensional and comprehensive diagnosis and treatment techniques of modern tumor medicine, TCM has been playing an irreplaceable and powerful role in the clinical treatment of tumors, and becoming more and more well known and recognized. After the 2018 Nobel Prize in Physiology or Medicine has been awarded, the immunotherapy for cancer is expected to be the most promising mean to cure cancer at present. However, due to the complexity, multidirectivity and uncontrollability of related immunodrugs in clinical pharmacological experiments, the immunotherapy still has many problems to be solved, such as the recurrence possibility and toxic reaction of CAR-T, PD-1, etc. resulting in limited clinical audiences and long-term efficacy, and the drugresistance of immunotherapy and the high cost are also problems that can not be ignored. At the

习近平总书记曾经说过:"中医药学凝聚着深邃的哲学智慧和中华民族几千年的健康养生理念及其实践经验,是中国古代科学的瑰宝,也是打开中华文明宝库的钥匙。深入研究和科学总结中医药学对丰富世界医学事业、推进生命科学研究具有积极意义。""医之为道大矣,医之为任重矣",从 1700 多年前先人葛洪在《肘后备急方》中记载"青蒿一握""绞取汁,尽服之"到第一位荣获诺贝尔生理学或医学奖的华人科学家屠呦呦女士成功研制出挽救数百万人生命的青蒿素,我们得以更加坚定地相信中医药赋予了现代医学以前沿性和颠覆性这一事实。

有鉴于此,本概述尝试从现代临床医学 I 级预防在癌前介入的具体实施与理论架构入手,以中医临床经典《伤寒论》的理、法、方、药为核心启发与切入点,并充分结

same time, the innovative opportunities and unique advantages brought about to TCM begin to take root and sprout at an unknown rate.

General Secretary Xi Jinping once said: "The TCM condenses profound philosophical wisdom and thousands of years of healthy ideas and practical experience of the Chinese nation, it is not only the treasure of ancient Chinese science, but also the key to open the treasure house of Chinese civilization. The intensive research and scientific summary of TCM are of positive significance to enrich the cause of world medicine and promote life science research." "Medicine is a great way, and the responsibilities of medicine are so heavy". Inspired by Ge Hong, an ancestor who recorded "squeeze the juice of a hold of artemisia apiacea and take it all" into *Zhouhou Beiji Fang* more than 1700 years ago, Ms. Tu Youyou has become the first Chinese scientist who won the Nobel Prize in Physiology or Medicine for successfully developing the artemisinin which has saved millions of lives. It makes us more firmly believe that the TCM endows the modern medicine with its frontier and overwhelming superiority.

In view of this, this outline attempts to start with the concrete implementation and theoretical framework of the grade I prevention of modern clinical medicine in the precancerous intervention, take the theory, method,

合后世各家学派与现代医学病生理学有关方面的内容，为广大肿瘤临床医学工作者提供有创新价值与临床意义的理论探索与临证启发，以期为现代临床肿瘤治疗提升整体防治能力，降低发病率、死亡率与癌患的生存负担提供一套切实有效的系统方案。

prescription and medicine of TCM as the core inspiration and entry point, and fully draw experience from the later TCM generations' theory and modern pathophysiology, to provide theoretical exploration and clinical enlightenment of innovative value and clinical significance for the majority of tumor clinical workers, so as to provide a set of practical and effective systematic schemes for modern clinical tumor treatment to improve the overall prevention and treatment ability and reduce the incidence, mortality and survival burden of cancer patients.

一、癌前病变的相关基础概念

目前学术界公认的癌症的经典发生与演变过程主要包括"正常上皮→单纯增生→异型增生→原位癌→浸润癌"。现代病理学认为从正常细胞发展为恶性肿瘤常常需要数年到数十年不等,一般从异型增生开始,细胞和组织的结构与功能开始发生明显改变,从而致使机体的整体病理态势向癌变方向发展,而在恶性肿瘤发生前的阶段则被称为癌前病变。所有的恶性肿瘤都有癌前病变,但并非所有的癌前病变都会发展为恶性肿瘤。致癌因素若持续存在,可最终导致恶性肿瘤的发生,倘若采取有效的干预与介入手段及时去除相关致癌因素,便可以使机体恢复到正常状态,摆脱癌变的可能。

由于恶性肿瘤的极端隐匿性与诊疗逃避性,使得常规临床接诊的绝大部分癌患已处于中晚期阶段,加之恶性肿瘤的猛烈性与破坏性,使得患者整体呈现预后不良趋势,而伴随的医疗难度与负担亦随之加大,这种极端反差与表

I.The Basic Concepts Related to Precancerous Lesions

At present, the classical occurrence and evolution of cancer which are recognized by academic circles mainly include "normal epithelium→simple hyperplasia→dysplasia→cancer in situ→infiltrating carcinoma". The modern pathology holds that it often takes years to decades for the development of normal cells to malignant tumors. Generally, the structure and function of cells and tissues begin to change obviously from dysplasia, which leads to the development of the overall pathological situation of the body to the direction of carcinogenesis, and the stage before the occurrence of malignant tumor is called precancerous lesion. All the malignant tumors have precancerous lesions, but not all precancerous lesions develop into malignant tumors. If the carcinogenic factors persist, they will lead to the occurrence of malignant tumor, but if effective intervention is taken to remove the related carcinogenic factors in time, the body will return to its normal state and get rid of the possibility of canceration.

Due to the extreme hiding and the diagnosis and treatment avoidance of the malignant tumor, the majority of the cancer patients in the routine clinical diagnosis have been in the middle and late stage. And because of the violent and destructive nature of the malignant tumor, the overall

现使癌症成为现代医学一直难以逾越的鸿沟，也是现代医学工作者研究与突破的热点。正如中医经典《黄帝内经》所言："是故圣人不治已病治未病，不治已乱治未乱"，倘若在癌前阶段未给予充分与及时的干预与处理，待到恶性肿瘤发生时，"譬犹渴而穿井，斗而铸锥，不亦晚乎？"笔者认为，由于恶性肿瘤特殊属性所带动的癌前病变兼具持续性与可逆性的发展过程，早期发现癌前病变与癌前介入将是降低恶性肿瘤死亡率、提升人类生命质量的根本途径与最佳切入点，也是现代肿瘤医学的核心突破点。

prognosis of the patients has shown a poor trend, and the accompanying medical difficulties and burdens have also increased. The extreme contrast and performance have made the cancer a difficult and insurmountable gap in modern medicine, and the cancer has also been a hot spot of the research and breakthrough for modern medical workers. As *Huangdi Neijing* contained: "Therefore, the sage usually pays less attention to the treatment of a disease, but more to the prevention". If adequate and timely intervention and treatment are not carried out in the precancerous phase until the malignant tumor occurs, "It's just like to dig a well when one feels thirsty and to cast a weapon when the war has already broken out. Isn't it too late?" The author thinks that the precancerous lesions driven by the specific properties of malignancies combining continuity and reversibility, and the early detection of precancerous lesions and precancerous intervention will be the fundamental approach and the best entry point of reducing the mortality of malignant tumors and improving the quality of human life, and will also be the core breakthrough point of modern tumor medicine.

二、癌前病变现代临床筛查与诊断的空缺

目前临床诊断早期肿瘤主要依靠医学影像学、细胞组织学和内镜初筛。病理学诊断是肿瘤学诊断的"金标准",也是医生进行临床治疗的依据。但患者往往是在具有明显的占位性病变后才得以确诊,从细胞癌变的生物学角度去理解,这种占位性病变已经不是癌变的最早期。癌前病变是一类隐蔽且复杂的组织学病理过程,几乎没有或极少见相应的临床表现。而由于目前常规使用的物理学、生物化学和病理学检查手段的限制,对癌前病变取材诊断、处理与研究极其困难。

常见的癌前病变筛查与诊断项目主要有粪便隐血试验、直肠指检、TCT、乳腺钼靶、B超、X线、胃镜、肠镜、肿瘤标志物联合检测等,但由于存在肿瘤标志物不敏感性与常规检查的诸多理论盲区和技术限制,使得大部分癌前阶段未被及时发现与介入治疗,许多患者在确诊恶性肿瘤之前的多年体检中也并未发现任何异常。可以说,现

II. The Defect of Modern Clinical Screening and Diagnosis of Precancerous Lesions

At present, clinical diagnosis of early tumors mainly depends on medical image, cell histology and endoscopic screening. Pathological diagnosis is the "gold standard" for oncology diagnosis, and it is also the basis for doctors to carry out clinical treatment. But patients are often diagnosed only after obvious space-occupying lesions, in the biological point of view of cell carcinogenesis, this kind of space-occupying lesion has not been the earliest stage of carcinogenesis. Precancerous lesions are a class of concealed and complex histopathological processes with little or no corresponding clinical manifestations. Due to the limitations of physical, biochemical and pathological examination methods, it is extremely difficult to diagnose, manage and study precancerous lesions.

The common items of screening and diagnosis of precancerous lesions are fecal occult blood test, digital rectal examination, TCT, breast mammography target, B-ultrasound, X-ray, gastroscopy, enteroscopy, combined detection of tumor markers and so on. However, due to the insensitivity of tumor markers, many theoretical blind areas and technical limitations of routine examinations, most of the precancerous stages have

代临床肿瘤学在癌前介入方面依然存在诸多不足与黑洞,充分汲取现代临床医学在肿瘤病理研究方面的成果,发挥中医学在"治未病"与宏观诊断、调控方面的巨大潜力与优势,是大势所趋,也是生命科学发展的必然。

not been found and treated in time. Many patients did not find any abnormalities in their physical examinations for many years before the definite diagnosis of malignant tumors. It can be said that there are still many shortcomings and black holes in modern clinical oncology in precancerous intervention. It is not only the trend of the times, but also the necessity of the development of life science to fully draw on the achievements of modern clinical medicine in tumor pathology research and to give full play to the great potential and advantages of TCM in "preventive treatment of disease", macroscopic diagnosis, and readjustment and control.

三、"柳暗花明又一村"——中医瞑眩反应介入的临床机理与诊疗优势

"瞑眩反应"是机体主动顺势疗法的临床主要表现形式,也是传统中医学独特的治疗经验。传统中医学认为每个人的自我修复能力是很强的,只不过现代医学过分关注疾病而非人体本身,局限的药物或手术的针对性治疗无法复制人体的自我修复能力,无法根据自身的能量大小、正气强弱来修复某些病变的地方。而我们即将介绍的瞑眩反应却恰恰弥补了现代医学在这方面的不足。

"瞑眩"一词最早来源于《尚书·说命上》:"若药不瞑眩,厥疾弗瘳。"日本古方派岱宗吉益东洞有云:"药毒也,而病毒也,药毒而攻病毒,所以瞑眩者也",如《伤寒杂病论》所载"初服微烦,复服汗出、如冒状及如醉状得吐、如虫行皮中、或血如豚肝、尿如皂汁、吐脓泻出之类","用之瞑眩,其毒从去,是仲景之为也"。近代中医泰斗岳美中先生亦曾经明确指出:"深痼之疾,服药中病则瞑眩,瞑眩愈剧,奏效愈宏。"日本汉方巨擘汤本求真

III. "There is a Way Out" — The Clinical Mechanism and the Diagnosis and Treatment Advantages of TCM in Dizziness Reaction Intervention

"Dizziness Reaction" is the main clinical manifestation of active homeopathic therapy, and it is also the unique treatment experience of TCM. The TCM holds that everyone's self-repair ability is very strong, it's just that modern medicine pays too much attention to the disease rather than the human body itself, and limited medicamentous or surgical targeted treatment cannot replicate the self-repair ability of the human body, and cannot repair some pathological changes according to patients' own energy size and the strength of healthy Qi. And the dizziness reaction we are about to introduce makes up for the shortcomings of modern medicine in this respect.

The word "Dizziness Reaction" first came from *Shang Shu*, a literature from ancient China — "If the person who is seriously ill or has a long-term illness takes the traditional Chinese medicine without having dizziness reaction, the patient won't recover." The ancient Japanese medical grandmaster Jiyi Dongdong once said: "Drugs are toxic, and the diseases are also toxic. The toxicity of drugs fights against the toxicity of diseases, which results in the dizziness reaction." As *Shanghan Zabing Lun* contained: "After taking the medicine, the patient feels uncomfortable,

亦曾于《皇汉医学》中载有《论中医治疗中瞑眩证状之发起者为原因疗法之确证》一文，读者亦可详参。

著名伤寒学者娄绍昆先生认为瞑眩反应的出现与《黄帝内经》中的反治法有着密不可分的临床联系。《黄帝内经》曰："微者逆之，甚者从之""正者正治，反者反治"。《黄帝内经》以朴素的文字形式表达了反治法的机制——把对主症的从治，纳入对病因、病证的逆治之中。这样，一方面能促进机体主体性反应，创造能充分显露主症的内

and the discomfort will be relieved after sweating. Or the patient feels dizzy and vomits like a drunk, feels like worms crawling under the skin, emits blood clots like cod liver, eliminates turbid urine like soap juice, vomits and excretes purulent fluid...after taking the medicine." Therefore, Jiyi Dongdong insisted: "The dizziness reaction that occurs after taking medicine causes the disease in the body to be cleared, which is the clinical characteristic of Chinese medical saint Zhang Zhongjing." The modern Chinese medicine master Yue Meizhong also made it clear that "The drug in the human body will cause the dizziness reaction if the disease is severe. The more violent the dizziness reaction is, the better the curative effect is." Japanese TCM master Tangben Qiuzhen also wrote *The Discussion on the Cause Therapy as the Confirmation of Generating Dizziness Reaction in TCM Treatment* in *Huang Han Medicine*, and the readers can also refer to the article in detail.

Lou Shaokun, a well-known specialist of *Shanghan Lun*, thinks that the occurrence of the dizziness reaction is closely related to the paradoxical treatment in *Huangdi Neijing*. As *Huangdi Neijing* contained: "Patients with weak disease elimination ability need treating contrary to their pathological manifestations, patients with strong disease elimination ability need treating according to their pathological manifestations" "Diseases conforming to the pathological dynamic need

环境，加强局部反馈信息，激活生理学上的"对抗系统"，促使邪正斗争由相持转向激化，当症状完全出来时，就能动摇机体的病理稳态而达到治愈疾病的目的。另一方面，又能最大限度地防止在从症治疗中，由于症状的加剧、病情的激化而造成的不良后果。

著名中医临床泰斗李可认为，瞑眩反应其机理缘于低一级时空的正常阴气与高一级时空的正常阳气相顺接刹那的反应。瞑眩现象出现一次，人体的能量提高一次，从某种角度讲是可遇不可求的事情。但临床实践也告知世人，并不是瞑眩现象出现的次数多，就肯定能取得明显疗效或

treating in a way conforming to the pathological dynamic; diseases contrary to the pathological dynamic need treating in a way contrary to the pathological dynamic", the *Huangdi Neijing* expresses the mechanism of paradoxical treatment in plain words — The essence of "paradoxical treatment" conforming pathological dynamic for the primary symptoms is still "explicable treatment" resisting pathological dynamic for the etiology and disease pattern. On the one hand, it can promote the subjective response of the body, create the internal environment that can fully reveal the main symptoms, highlight the partial feedback information, activate the antagonistic system of physiology, and facilitate the combat between healthy Qi and pathogenic Qi transforming from stalemate into intensified situation. When the symptoms come out completely, we can achieve the purpose of curing the disease by means of shaking the pathological homeostasis of the body. On the other hand, it can prevent the aggravation of symptoms and diseases in explicable treatment from causing adverse consequences furthest.

Li Ke, a famous clinical master of TCM, believes that the mechanism of dizziness reaction is due to the reaction of a split second when the normal Yin Qi in the lower order space-time and the normal Yang Qi in the higher order space-time are phase-connected. Each time when dizziness reaction occurs accompanying with one time when the energy of human

救人之命。中医是治病了的人,而人赖以生存的那口气时时刻刻在变化,能够驾驭这口气的是每个人自己的心而不是医者手中的术。

正如《道德经》所言:"将欲歙之,必故张之。将欲弱之,必故强之。将欲废之,必故兴之。将欲取之,必故与之。是谓微明。柔弱胜刚强。鱼不可脱于渊,国之利器不可以示人。"火神鼻祖郑钦安亦认为,凡服药后常有"变动",要知道这些变动有的是"药与病相攻者,病与药相拒者",属于正常的药物反应,"岂即谓药不对症乎?"

body increases. In a way, it's a rare and precious case. However, clinical practice also tells that the dizziness reaction occurring more often doesn't mean that the obvious curative effect or life saving can be achieved more promisingly. The one that TCM treats is the real person who is sick, and the Qi on which people depend for their survival is constantly changing, and it is everyone's own spirit instead of the technology in the hands of the healer that can control this Qi.

As *Dao De Jing*, a philosophical literature from ancient China, contained: "If you want to converge it, expand it first; If you want to weaken it, strengthen it first; If you want to abolish it, initiate it first; If you want to get it, give it first. All things in the world exist and change in this kind of subtle and clear form. This form is very mild, but there is no means to destroy it. The relationship between water and fish conforms to the regular pattern in the universe. The country's core weapon, the root of the country's survival, can't be shown to outsiders, which also conforms to." Zheng Qinan, the founder of the fire god school of TCM, believed that there are often "changes" after taking the medicine, the changes that "drugs and diseases attack and resist with each other" belong to the normal drug reactions. "How can we say that the medicine does not fit the disease?"

纵观《伤寒论》全书，"烦"字的出现频率极高，笔者认为，《伤寒论》中绝大多数"烦"应当为人体的一种明显的"瞑眩反应"程度表达抑或是正气来复或者邪气益甚的表现形式。结合临床对于"烦"字的深入体会，我们得以窥察到医圣张仲景对于"瞑眩"的认知过程与临证处理。

如《伤寒论》第24条"太阳病，初服桂枝汤，反烦不解者，先刺风池、风府，却与桂枝汤则愈"；

《伤寒论》第46条"服药已微除，其人发烦目瞑，剧者必衄，衄乃解"；

《伤寒论》第57条"伤寒发汗已解，半日许复烦"；

《伤寒论》第147条方后注"初服微烦，复服汗出便愈"；

In the whole of *Shanghan Lun*, the occurrence frequency of the word "Fan" is very high. The author believes that the vast majority of "Fan" in *Shanghan Lun* should be an obvious expression of the degree of "dizziness reaction" of the human body or a specific expression of recovery of healthy Qi or aggravation of pathogenic Qi. According to the clinical experience of the word "Fan", we can look through the cognitive process and clinical treatment of Chinese medical saint Zhang Zhongjing on the "dizziness reaction".

Such us article 24 of *Shanghan Lun* records: "Due to Taiyang disease, the patient took Cortex Cinnamon Decoction, in case that the patient felt 'Fan' and the disease had not been alleviated. In the circumstances, the patient should be given acupuncture at Fengchi and Fengfu and take Cortex Cinnamomi Decoction again, then the patient will be cured";

Article 46 of *Shanghan Lun* records: "After taking the medicine, the patient got better and immediately felt 'Fan' in case of a nosebleed, and then the disease will be relieved";

Article 57 of *Shanghan Lun* records: "The patient suffering from the Shanghan disease had been relieved after the sweating of the medicine and then felt 'Fan' a half day later";

The prescription notes under Article 147 of *Shanghan Lun* records: "The patient felt a little 'Fan' after taking the medicine, and then recovered after sweating caused by the next medication";

《伤寒论》第 289 条"时自烦,欲去衣被者,可治"等,

包括《伤寒论》第 94 条"太阳病未解,脉阴阳俱停,必先振栗汗出而解";

《伤寒论》第 98 条"与柴胡汤,后必下重";

《伤寒论》第 101 条"复与柴胡汤,必蒸蒸而振,却复发热汗出而解";

《伤寒论》第 174 条方后注"初一服,其人身如痹,半日许复服之,三服都尽,其人如冒状";

《伤寒论》第 192 条"小便反不利,大便自调,其人骨节疼,翕翕如有热状,奄然发狂,濈然汗出而解";

《伤寒论》第 243 条"得汤反剧者,属上焦也";

Article 289 of *Shanghan Lun* records: "When Shaoyin patient who has chills and curls himself up in bed feels 'Fan' and wants to remove his clothes and quilt, it is an indication of a curable case"; etc.

Including Article 94 of *Shanghan Lun* records: "After treatment, the patient did not recover as expected, the diagnosis showed that the patient's pulses both at Yang and Yin were comparable, and then the patient will recover through full of shivering with cold and sweating";

Article 98 of *Shanghan Lun* records: "After taking Bupleuri Decoction, the patient will then have diarrhea";

Article 101 of *Shanghan Lun* records: "If Bupleuri Decoction syndrome still exists, then the decoction can still be adopted. The patient then is feverish, shivers and perspires. And the syndrome is gone at the same time";

The prescription notes under Article 174 of *Shanghan Lun* records: "After taking the first dose, the patient will have a sensation of numbness. And half a day later, the patient takes the second dose. When the three doses are finished, the patient will become dizzy";

Article 192 of *Shanghan Lun* records: "The patient had normal stools, but had dysuria. And the bone joint was algesic accompanied by a mild fever, then the patient suddenly went mad, recovered through sweating ceaselessly";

Article 243 of *Shanghan Lun* records: "The vomiting

《伤寒论》第278条"系在太阴,太阴当发身黄……至七八日,虽暴烦下利日十余行,必自止,以脾家实,腐秽当去故也"等。

这些条文,都充分彰显了张仲景作为"医圣"异于常人的临证思维与分析处理能力,也正是这些可贵之处的启发,为我们从伤寒六经层面深度剖析瞑眩反应的临床机制与应对原则提供了切实可行的切入点。

综合上述相关分析,笔者尝试从现代医学角度对瞑眩反应作出如下定义:

瞑眩反应是指病理状态下的个体在药物以及其他治疗方式的良性诱导下建立起的一种抗损伤和修复能力的表现,是一种打破病理稳态、重新构筑人体免疫新平衡的发生过程,也是诸多慢性痼疾治愈过程的中心环节。主要表现为急性炎症与良性应激的有规律发生。治疗方向准确的

of the patient intensified after taking medicine, which was due to the excretion of cold fluid-retention in upper energizer membrane";

Article 278 of *Shanghan Lun* records: "The condition of the disease is in the Taiyin, and the patient of Taiyin disease should have Yin icterus...By the seventh or eighth day, the diarrhea which suddenly appeared more than ten times a day would have stopped naturally. This is because the body is full of healthy Qi, and the endotoxins of the body are excreted out"; etc.

These articles excerpted above fully show up Zhang Zhongjing's fantastic clinical thinking and handling capacity as "Chinese medical saint", and also provide practical and feasible entry point for us to deeply analyze the clinical mechanism and coping principles of the dizziness reaction from the level of six meridians in *Shanghan Lun*.

Based on the relevant analysis above, the author tries to define the dizziness reaction from the perspective of modern medicine as follows:

The Dizziness Reaction refers to the expression of anti-injury and repair ability established by individuals in pathological state under the benign induction of drugs and other methods of treatment. It is a process of breaking pathological homeostasis and reconstructing the new balance of human immunity, and it is also the key link in the treatment

话可能会激发体内潜伏已久的邪气外托，加之药物以及其他治疗方式促进正气来复，正邪得以交争，人体自然会产生相应的排邪反应，也就是促进了免疫应答和正向代偿反应。

由于瞑眩反应与急性炎症以及良性应激的特殊关联性，很多患者会因中药免疫治疗导致免疫细胞释放出大量刺激性化学物质，产生皮肤、呼吸系统、消化系统或泌尿生殖系统的相关反应。

例如笔者的一位心肌梗死引发急性左心衰的男性患者，在服用大回阳通脉茯苓四逆汤合甘遂半夏汤后，于左胸手厥阴心包经循行处透发大量紫黑色疱疹，笔者为之刺络拔罐放血，针药结合治疗20余天后患者恢复常态。

of many chronic and difficult diseases. The main manifestations are the regular occurrences of Acute Inflammation and Eustress. If the treatment direction is accurate, it could stimulate the pathogenic Qi that has been lurking in the body for a long time to be expelled. In addition, the drugs and other methods of treatment can promote the recovery of healthy Qi so that the healthy Qi can fight against with the pathogenic Qi adequately, and the human body will naturally produce the corresponding "exorcism reaction" — It will promote the immune response and the positive compensation reaction.

Owing to the special relationship among Dizziness Reaction, Acute Inflammation and Eustress, many patients will release a large number of irritating chemicals from immune cells due to the immunotherapy of TCM, resulting in the related reactions of skin, respiratory system, digestive system or genitourinary system.

For example, one of the author's male patients with acute left heart failure caused by myocardial infarction, after taking Dahuiyang Tongmai Fuling Sini Decoction and Euphorbia Kansui Pinellia Ternata Decoction, there were a large number of purple and black herpes appearing in Jueyin pericardium meridian of hand on the left chest. Then the author gave him acupuncture, cupping and bloodletting, and the patient recovered after more than 20 days of acupuncture and TCM treatment.

再如笔者的一位代谢综合征女性患者，在服用中药免疫处方5剂后就随之出现了全腹剧烈的绞痛，当地医院检查发现患者腹内出现渗出性脓液，在笔者的说服下患者放弃了外科手术，后处以大陷胸汤加减化裁而治愈。

无独有偶，娄绍昆先生亦曾遇到过相似的案例：李某，女，45岁，胃中不适用半夏泻心汤治疗。服药后有效，遂守原方，2个月治疗后胃中不适消失，但是月经淋漓不止。因服药前从未有过此情况，患者坚持认为这是医疗事故，不依不饶。考虑再三，让她去做全面的检查，检查后发现是宫颈癌。

又如国内科学家陈小平与钟南山院士作为共同研究者经历了14年的机理探讨发现疟原虫感染可能激活人体的天然或获得性免疫系统从而对癌细胞产生了一定的杀伤效果。而目前正在开展的通过人为诱导肺癌患者出现疟疾而产生定向免疫从而依靠人体主动性杀死自身肿瘤细胞的医

Another example is that one of the author's female patients with metabolic syndrome appeared severe colic in the whole abdomen after taking 5 doses of immunization prescription of TCM. The local hospital examination found some exudative pus in the abdomen of the patient. Under the persuasion of the author, the patient gave up the surgery and was cured with the addition of Daxianxiong Decoction.

Similarly, Lou Shaokun has encountered similar cases: Ms. Li, 45 years old, felt uncomfortable in the stomach, Dr. Lou prescribed her Pinellia Ternata Xiexin Decoction, and the patient felt better after taking the decoction, so Dr. Lou continued to prescribe her original decoction. After 2 months of treatment, the discomfort of patient's stomach disappeared, but the patient had prolonged menstruation. Because there had never been such a situation before taking the medicine, the patient insisted that it was a medical accident and blamed to Dr. Lou. On second thought, Dr. Lou asked her to have a full physical examination and eventually she was diagnosed with cervical cancer.

Likewise, Chinese scientist Chen Xiaoping and Academician Zhong Nanshan, as co-researchers, have been studying the mechanism of Plasmodium falciparum infection for 14 years and found that Plasmodium falciparum infection may activate the natural or acquired immune system of human body and have a certain killing effect on cancer cells. And

学研究亦方兴未艾。

再如中国中医科学院西苑医院通过临床试验研究发现"扶助阳气,促使阳气旺盛,阳气与毒邪由相持转向激化,则可能缩短病程,促使慢性肝炎的恢复"。由此可见,当慢性病处于功能代偿、代谢代偿阶段,治疗时如能产生瞑眩,出现一时性的症状加重、化验指标阳性及定量值上升,甚至出现部分组织坏死等情况,却能获得痊愈。

通过以上5个案例的系统分析,并结合笔者个人的临证经验,笔者在此尝试总结出瞑眩反应最基本的两个作用:

一是起疾病预测与鉴别诊断作用。传统的中医诊断并不是万能的,而通过瞑眩反应所打破的病理稳态进行疾病预测与诊断恰恰能帮助我们弥补在传统诊断上的不足,甚至相

the medical research about producing targeted immunity by artificially inducing malaria in patients with lung cancer to kill their own cancer cells relying on the initiative of the human body be just unfolding.

What's more, through clinical trials, the Xiyuan Hospital of China Institute of TCM found that "It is possible to shorten the course of disease and promote the recovery of chronic hepatitis by stimulating and flourishing Yang Qi to make the interaction between Yang Qi and poison evil change from stalemate to intensified situation". Thus it can be seen that when the chronic diseases are in the stage of functional compensation and metabolic compensation, if the dizziness reaction is able to occur during treatment resulting in the temporary aggravation of symptoms, positive laboratory indexes, increased quantitative values, even the necrosis of some tissues, etc., the chronic diseases may have the possibilities to be cured instead.

According to the systematic analysis of the five cases discussed above and personal clinical experience, the author tries to sum up the two most basic functions of dizziness reaction:

First, it plays a role in predicting disease and differential diagnosis. The TCM diagnosis is not universal, and the disease prediction and diagnosis through the pathological homeostasis broken by dizziness reaction can help us to make up for the

比现代西医学的诊断而言，这种诊断更具实用性和临床指导性。笔者认为，现代医学束手无策的阿尔茨海默症或许也可以在瞑眩反应的疾病预测与防治方面找到一些启发。

二是起直接治疗作用。瞑眩反应本身就是一种排病诱导，实际上类似于一种免疫活化过程，很多慢性痼疾的治愈靠的就是这个过程。

可以说，瞑眩反应是中医相较于西医所特有的诊疗优势，也是中医"不治已病治未病"与"揆度奇恒"的深刻体现。

shortcomings of the routine diagnosis. And it is even more practical and directional than the modern diagnosis. The author believes that we might also find some inspiration in the prediction and prevention of dizziness reaction for the study of Alzheimer's disease which is helpless in modern medicine.

Second, it has the effect of direct treatment. Dizziness reaction itself is a kind of induction of disease-removing. It is actually similar to the immune activation process, and it is the pivotal process in which many chronic and difficult diseases are cured.

It can be said that the dizziness reaction is the unique diagnosis and treatment advantage of TCM compared with modern medicine, and it is also the profound embodiment of "preventive treatment of disease" and "general and particular differentiation" in TCM theories.

四、中医辨证观下癌前阶段的常见特征性病理表现

由于现代医学尚未明确给出系统而又完整的癌前阶段常见特征性病理表现,为了便于一般临床筛查与向患者临床普及,笔者尝试结合传统中医六经辨证与现代临床医学综合症候群的思想,将规律性与典型性较强且易于常规诊察的病理表现总结如下:

一定阶段内不明原因的体重明显大幅度下降;

气力不足,易疲易乏;
半夜易醒,醒后或伴有盗汗;

周身骨节肌肉常伴有固定性酸楚疼痛,且常规外治方式缓解不明显或反复发作难愈,以少阳经循行处为典型;

肩颈后背常伴有固定性酸楚疼痛,且与气候变迁及寒热变化有明显关联性;

IV. Common Characteristic Pathological Manifestations of Precancerous Stage under the View of Syndrome Differentiation in TCM

Modern medicine has not clearly presented systematic and complete common characteristic pathological manifestations in precancerous stage. In order to facilitate general clinical screening and precancerous popularization to patients, the author tries to sum up the pathological manifestations with strong regularity and typicality and easily diagnosed by routine examination referring to the idea of six-meridian syndrome differentiation of TCM and syndrome of modern clinical medicine as follows:

Losing the weight of body significantly of unknown reason in a certain period;

Feeling hypodynamic and easy to get tired obviously;

Waking up frequently in the middle of the night accompanied by night sweat possibly;

Having fixed discomfort and pain which are recurrent, difficult to be cured by routine external treatment, and mainly distributed in Shaoyang meridians at bones and muscles all over the body;

Having fixed discomfort and pain which are significantly related to climate and temperature changes at shoulder, neck and back;

病理性汗出异常（汗出部位异常、汗出量异常）；

大便持续性异常（形状异常、颜色异常），频率偏低（数日不大便）或偏高（一日排便三次以上）；

半夜口干口黏严重；

晨起口苦明显；
口渴而不欲饮；
头面部易频繁上火；

异常耳鸣或鼻塞且持续时间较长；

咽喉有梗阻或异物感，常规检查无异常；

长期咳嗽不愈，甚引胸胁疼痛；

身体突然出现异常肿物或皮疹；

午后或夜间容易手足发热；

常年不感冒或频繁感冒；
感冒一次如同大病一场，需要很长时间恢复；

Having abnormal pathological sweat which involves site and amount;

Having persistent and abnormal stools which involves shape, color and frequency (astriction for a few days or defecation more than three times a day);

Having obvious and frequent dry or viscous sense in mouth in the middle of the night;

Having obvious bitter taste in mouth in the morning;

Feeling thirsty but unwilling to drink;

Having discomforts related to "the fire characterized by flaring up" such as inflammation occurring frequently in the part above the neck;

Having abnormal tinnitus or nasal congestion which lasts for a long time;

Having the sense of obstruction or foreign matter in the throat that has not been found abnormal in routine diagnosis;

Suffering a cough that has not been cured for a long time and even causes pain in chest and hypochondrium;

Having abnormal masses or rashes that occur suddenly on the body;

Having a fever appearing obviously after noon or at night in hands or feet;

Having no or frequent colds all year round;

Catching a cold like suffering a serious illness which takes a long time to cure;

持续性烦躁与疲劳；
嗜食大量生、冷、水果；
长期吸烟、饮酒、熬夜；
食用辛辣等厚味食物或不洁食物后不易出现腹泻；

长期反酸、腹胀、腹痛；

情绪思维突然异于常态，性格突变；
长期压抑阴郁，意欲不振；

性格偏激或怪异无常；
舌下或舌侧瘀络瘀点明显；

舌正中裂痕深而长；
舌苔厚腻色异常或水滑少苔、无苔；

脉位较沉，常规中取摸不到；

持续出现双脉或孕脉后排除患者受孕；

脉象含义与患者体征明显不符；

面布水斑，面色阴暗；

胸口或心下长期痞闷不适；

Having persistent anxiety and fatigue;

Being fond of eating a lot of raw food, cold food and fruit;

Smoking, drinking and staying up late over a long period of time;

Having infrequent occurrence of diarrhea after eating heavy taste or unclean food;

Having long-term acid regurgitation, abdominal distension and pain;

Appearing sudden change of character;

Having long-term depression of gloom and loss of motivation;

Being extreme or weird in character;

Having obvious blood stasis collaterals or points under or on the side of the tongue;

Having deep and long cracks on the middle of the tongue;

Having greasy, curdy, abnormal-color, slippery or sparse coating on the tongue;

Having the hidden pulse which is not easily diagnosed in the position of deep level;

Having continuous occurrence of double or pregnant pulse without pregnancy;

Having the pulse with meaning which is obviously inconsistent with the physical state;

Having the face which is dark and covered with water spots;

Suffering a long time discomfort of stuffiness in chest or

脐周条索状物或结节明显或出现腹直正中芯；

心下、脐上、脐下动悸较明显；

少腹急结；

局部炎症反复迁延难以愈合。

需要注意的是，以上所列症状在癌前病变群体中并非单独出现，临证诊察应以伤寒六经少阳、少阴病理为铃，当患者出现上述较多指证时，即可高度怀疑为癌前病变，病理稳态严重者甚至已经进入癌症阶段（即病理次第进一步内陷太阴、厥阴），此时实验室及影像学检查即可确诊，而此时患者的部分副癌综合征或单一临床表现也容易与上述症状相混淆，因此现代医学检查的介入在我们的体系中也是十分必要的。

epigastrium;

Having nodes around the navel or pencil-like nodes in the middle of the hypogastrium;

Having the beating of abdominal aorta around epigastrium, umbilical region and hypogastrium, which can be detected obviously in palpation;

Having spasmatic pain in lateral lower abdomen during abdominal palpation;

Having partial inflammation which is difficult to cure for a long time.

It should be noted that the symptoms summarized above do not appear alone in the precancerous lesion population, and the clinical diagnosis should be guided by the pathology of Shaoyang and Shaoyin. When the patients significantly have a few symptoms summarized above and are diagnosed with Shaoyang and Shaoyin diseases, they can be highly suspected to have precancerous lesions. The patients with severe pathological homeostasis have even entered the stage of cancer — The pathological level further invades Taiyin and Jueyin. At this time, the cancer can be diagnosed through laboratory and imageology examinations. Because some of the paracancerous syndromes or single clinical manifestations of the patients are easily confused with the symptoms summarized above, the intervention of modern medical examination is also very necessary in our clinical system.

五、中医辨证观下癌前病变病因的探讨

癌前病变的发生,多由长期烦劳过度、内伤七情、生活不节而致正气内虚、气血津液代谢失常,致使邪毒逐渐羁留胶踞成巢,久之积损成患,影响人体脏腑的正常职司功能并进一步损伤人体正气,如此形成长期恶性循环,最终酿生难以逆转之恶性致命病变。

癌前病变是现代西方医学病理研究的新兴领域,然而早在两千多年前我们的祖先便对此有了清晰而又深刻的认识。《黄帝内经》就曾有云:"血海有余,则常想其身大,怫然不知其所病;血海不足,亦常想其身小,狭然不知其所病。"这里的"血海"代指的是人体的双向应激功能与正负代偿状态;"身大"与"身小"并非特指患者的身材体格,而是代指"少阳"与"少阴"两种不同枢机下病理过渡的体质属性;"怫然"与"狭然"则暗示了大多数患

V. Discussion on the Etiology of Precancerous Lesions under the View of Syndrome Differentiation in TCM

The occurrence of precancerous lesions is mostly caused by excessive anxiety and fatigue for a long time, internal injury of seven feelings and disorderly life, bringing about deficiency of healthy Qi and abnormal metabolism of Qi, blood and body fluids, leading to the result that pathogenic toxins detain stubbornly into "nests" gradually. The long-term accumulation of damage caused by the "nests" can affect the normal function of Zang-fu organs and further damage the healthy Qi of the human body, thus it forms a long-term vicious circle which ultimately leads to malignant and fatal lesions that can not be reversed.

Precancerous state is a new field of modern pathology research, but as early as two thousand years ago, our ancestors had a clear and profound understanding of it. As *Huangdi Neijing* contained: "The sufficient blood sea leads to the big condition and arrogance without knowing the disease of oneself; the insufficient blood sea leads to the small condition and narrowness without knowing the disease of oneself." The "blood sea" mentioned above refers to the two-way stress function and the positive-negative compensation state of the human body; the "big condition" and "small condition" do

者处于癌前病变过程中最普遍的基本状态——身体并无明显不适。而正是由于恶性肿瘤这种隐匿恶变过程极不易被人察觉，所以当前临床中有近七成的恶性肿瘤患者在确诊后已濒临中晚期状态，此时医生的干预治疗以及患者的整体预后不甚理想。

长期从事临床的医师或许可以发现：许多慢性病缠身需要长期服药与疗养的患者的整体生存长度并非不理想，最终"带疾终天"的老年人数见不鲜；而又有很多平时看上去非常健康不易患病的人却会突然遭受一些看似出人意料的重大疾病，甚则死亡。所以，笔者认为，容易患病与否与是否真正健康并无太大关联，一个人的自我代偿功能与良性修复过程才是判断其生命质量好坏的标准。

not refer specifically to the stature of the patient, but to the constitutions of the pathological transitions under the different pivots of "Shaoyang" and "Shaoyin"; the "arrogance" and "narrowness" suggest that most patients who are in the most common basic state of precancerous lesions don't have any obvious discomfort. And it is precisely because the hidden malignant transformation process of malignant tumor is very difficult to be detected, nearly 70% of the malignant tumor patients are on the verge of middle and advanced state after diagnosis. At this time, the intervention treatments and the overall prognosis of the patients are very hopeless.

The doctors who have been engaged in clinic for a long time may find that the overall survival length of many chronic patients who need long-term medication and recuperation is not unideal as we expected and the elderly people who prolong life with disease are not uncommon. However, many people who usually look very healthy and not easy to get sick suddenly suffer from seemingly unexpected severe disease and even die on it. Therefore, the author believes that whether it is easy to get sick or not has little to do with whether it is really healthy or not, a person's self-compensation function and benign repair process are the criteria to judge the quality of life.

六、中医辨证观下癌前病变病位的探讨

三焦膜腠是癌前病变最主要的病位。笔者认为，三焦膜腠类似于人体全身的浆膜、黏膜以及细胞组织之间的间隙等，相当于人体全身的膜结构系统，也是中医体系中最大的免疫组织，是致病因子入侵、蓄积与转移的主要场所。"肥甘无度""肝气郁结""阳虚水泛""湿瘀互结""正气失司""伏邪成巢"等都会导致三焦枢机不利，进而引起或加重人体气、血、津液代谢障碍。

三焦膜腠的概念与刘完素在《素问玄机原病式》中提出的"玄府气液宣通"理论极为相似。中医经典《黄帝内经》中认为玄府为汗孔，而刘完素认为"玄府者，无物不有，人之脏腑、皮毛、肌肉、筋膜、骨髓、爪牙，至于世之万物，尽皆有之，乃气升降出入运行之道路门户也"，即玄府是人体各种组织腠理的统称，为人体气液运行之

VI. Discussion on the Location of Precancerous Lesions under the View of Syndrome Differentiation in TCM

The triple energizer membrane is the most important location of the precancerous lesions. The author thinks that the triple energizer membrane seems to be the interval between serosa, mucosa and the cell tissue. It is equivalent to the whole membrane structure system of the human body, and is also the largest immune organization in TCM system and the main place for invasion, accumulation and transfer of pathogenic factors. The unrestrained diet of junk food, stagnation of liver Qi, water diffusion due to deficiency of Yang, combination of phlegm and blood stasis, exhaustion of healthy Qi, "nests" stubbornly formed by latent evils, etc. can lead to the confused functions of the triple energizer membrane which further causes or aggravates the metabolic disorder of the Qi, blood and body fluids in the human body.

The concept of the triple energizer membrane is extremely similar to the theory of "Qi-fluids communication in 'mysterious mansion'" put forward in *Exploration to Mysterious Pathogenesis and Etiology Based on the Plain Questions* by Liu Wansu, the head of the four great physicians of the Jin and Yuan period. The "mysterious mansion" is interpreted as the sweat hole in *Huangdi Neijing*, and Liu Wansu held the point that "The 'mysterious mansion'

通道，与中医理论中的"通会元真之处"、藏医理论中的"水脉"有着异曲同工之妙。

而2018年在 Scientific Reports 刊载报道的之前从未见过的充满液体的空间网络组织——"间质"亦与中医的三焦膜腠吻合度极高，这种"间质"存在于皮肤表层下方，用来连接动脉、静脉、肌肉筋膜、肠道、肺等所有器官和组织，类似于一个极其精微、充满液体、涵盖并穿透结缔组织的通道网，相当于人体器官组织间液体流动的"高速公路"，遍布全身。

与许多脏腑器官不同，三焦膜腠本身独特的位置结构与功能属性，导致了其发病的牵连波及性、病能多变性与病变复杂性。由于三焦膜腠为"水道""决渎之官"，亦即人体津液代谢的通路，人体的气化失常则会导致津液的代谢与输布失常，从而导致津液停聚、滥溢或损耗，前二者

is everywhere, and it consists in the Zang-fu organs, fur, muscles, anadesma, bones and even other creatures' bodies, and it is the main thoroughfare and door for the ascending, descending, exiting and entering of Qi" — It shows that the "mysterious mansion" is the general term of the interstitium, and it is also the channel for the operations of Qi, blood and body fluids. Besides, the "mysterious mansion" is aiso similar to "the place where true origin operates" in the theory of TCM and the "water vessel" in the theory of Tibetan medicine.

The interstitium, a liquid-filled space network that has never been seen before in the human body and is reported in 2018 in *Scientific Reports*, also has a high degree of coincidence with the triple energizer membrane of TCM. This interstitium exists below the surface of the skin and is used to connect all organs and tissues, such as arteries, veins, muscle fascia, intestines and lungs. It is similar to very small and liquid-filled of channel networks that cover and penetrate the connective tissue. And we can compare it to the "highway" of liquid flowing between organs and tissues all over the body.

Unlike many of the Zang-fu organs, the unique position structure and function property of the triple energizer membrane have led to the implicated spread, pathological complexity and the changeability of the disease. The triple energizer membrane which is referred to as the "water pathway" and "organ official in charge of dredging" in *Huangdi Neijing* is the pathway of body

可以衍生为"湿""痰""痞""浊""瘀"等有形之邪而导致诸多变证，后者则会导致虚损证候的出现。

有形之邪的长期郁滞，加之旁系疾病的诱发与并发，可导致类似于《伤寒论》"结胸""脏结"等严重后果，患者往往会表现为"憋闷感""窒息感""梗阻感"与"胀痛感"。由于三焦膜腠为相火之本府，有形之阴邪的长期郁闭亦可导致相火怫郁不得宣达，由此而化热化火甚至逆乱妄动，同时加之现代不良生活方式而导致的通会元真水道之真阳的耗损与不足，患者势必会呈现出寒热虚实错综复杂之象——阴邪郁遏在内、相火妄生邪热、阳气卫外不足的水火相争之格局，随之亦会加大临床诊治的难度。恶性肿瘤之所以棘手难治，亦由于此。

fluids metabolism. The disorders of Qi transformation can lead to the disharmony of the body fluids metabolism, which can result in the accumulation, overflow or loss of the body fluids. The first two can be derived as tangible pathological products such as dampness, phlegm, focal distention, turbidity and accumulated stasis, which can lead to numerous deteriorative syndromes. And the last one can cause deficiency syndromes.

Tangible pathological products' long-term depression and stagnation combined with the induction and concurrency of collateral diseases can lead to serious consequences such as "thoracic accumulation" and "binding of Zang-viscera" in *Shanghan Lun*, and the patients often have senses of oppression, suffocation, obstruction and distending pain. Because the triple energizer membrane is the house of ministerial fire in TCM theory, the long-term depression and stagnation of tangible pathological products can also lead to the restraint and even frenetic stirring of ministerial fire. And because the consumption and deficiency of true Yang in the triple energizer membrane due to the unhealthy modern life style, the patients are bound to appear the complex images of cold-heat and deficiency-excess, a pattern of fire and water combat caused by pathological products depressed inside, the internal blaze of ministerial fire and the deficient assignment of Yang Qi in external. Thus, the difficulty of clinical diagnosis and treatment has been increased evidently. Based on the analysis above, we can imagine how difficult it is to treat malignant tumors.

七、中医辨证观下癌前病变病机的探讨

"少阳、少阴失枢,太阴阴盛阳衰"是癌前病变的核心病机。

《黄帝内经》有云:"三阳之离合也,太阳为开,阳明为阖,少阳为枢;三阴之离合也,太阴为开,厥阴为阖,少阴为枢。"少阴病与少阳病在《伤寒论》中的地位很特殊,从整个地球和人类的进化史来看,我们现在应该处于少阳与少阴交界过渡的时期,整个地球或人类社会的演进的确已经到达中年,甚至是中晚年的阶段。为了方便读者系统理解《伤寒论》六经的动态演变过程,笔者结合个人创作的 The Six Channels Samsara 曲线略做分析:

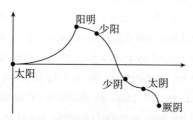

The Six Channels Samsara 曲线

VII. Discussion on the Pathogenesis of Precancerous Lesions under the View of Syndrome Differentiation in TCM

The disorders of pivots in Shaoyang and Shaoyin and the exuberance of Yin with decline of Yang in Taiyin are the core pathogenesises of precancerous lesions.

As *Huangdi Neijing* contained: "As to the separation and combination of three Yang, Taiyang is responsible for opening, Yangming for closing and Shaoyang for pivoting; As to the separation and combination of three Yin, Taiyin is responsible for opening, Jueyin for closing and Shaoyin for pivoting." The Shaoyin and Shaoyang diseases play extremely special roles in *Shanghan Lun*. Judging from the evolution history of the whole earth and human beings, we should now be in a period of transition between Shaoyang and Shaoyin. The evolution of the whole earth or human society has indeed reached the stage of middle and old age. In order to facilitate readers to systematically understand the dynamic evolution of the six meridians in *Shanghan Lun*, the author tries to make a brief analysis referring to The Six Channels Samsara Curve created by himself:

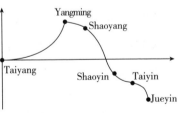

The Six Channels Samsara Curve

首先,《黄帝内经》中的"离合"代指生命朴素而又终极的奥秘——生死相续,如环无端,二者共同构成了完整的生命过程。"开"者,代指原始生命大潮动荡之开启,此动荡暗含生化、衰败二势,动荡之剧取决于曲线之斜率（K）;"阖"者,代指原始生命大潮动荡之极尽,此动荡暗含生化、衰败二势,动荡之剧取决于曲线之斜率（K）;"枢"者,代指原始生命大潮阴阳巨变之转承,此动荡暗含阴阳离合二势,动荡之剧取决于曲线之斜率（K）。

太阳作为初生之一阳,是生命之始;阳明为"两阳合明",多气多血,乃阳之最旺。太阳犹如"星星之火",倘若顾护得当,大有阳明"燎原"之态势。从太阳至阳明对应的生理年龄段主要集中在童年、少年时期,在此期间的病理表现多集中于急性病,如高热、肺炎、急性肠胃炎、川崎病、猩红热、痘疹等。

少阳本身极具迷幻色彩,因其病位广泛而又界限模

First of all, the "separation and combination" in *Huangdi Neijing* refer to the simple and ultimate mystery of life — Life and death continue each other, just like an endless loop, which forms a complete life process. The "opening" refers to the beginning of the transformation of the wave of primitive life, which implies the tendencies of exuberance and debilitation, and the intensity of the transformation depends on the slope of the curve (K); The "closing" refers to the end of the transformation of the wave of primitive life, which implies the tendencies of exuberance and debilitation, and the intensity of the transformation depends on the slope of the curve (K); The "pivoting" refers to the pivot of the transformation of the wave of primitive life, which implies the tendencies of division and unity of Yin and Yang, and the intensity of the transformation depends on the slope of the curve (K).

As the newborn one, Taiyang is the beginning of life; Yangming is the two-yang unity full of Qi and blood, and is the most prosperous Yang. Taiyang is like "a single spark", if taken good care of, there will be "a prairie fire" in Yangming. The corresponding physiological age group from Taiyang to Yangming mainly focuses on children and teenager, during which the pathological manifestations are more concentrated in acute diseases, such as high fever, pneumonia, acute gastroenteritis, Kawasaki disease, scarlatina and rash.

Shaoyang itself is extremely psychedelic. It can communicate

糊，可沟通表里上下阴阳，故喜清泄宣通为用、恶郁结凝聚为碍。从阳明至少阳对应的生理年龄段主要集中在青少年、青壮年时期，阳性渐收，阴性渐生，理智与感性逐渐趋于协调，身体不但要迎合少阳春生之发陈，更要适应灵魂生长成熟之节奏，倘若不迎合此态势，则易变生少阳相火妄动或闭阻郁结之态势，从而诱发植物神经紊乱、焦虑症、甲亢、消化道溃疡、胆囊炎、心肌炎、肺结核、鼻咽炎、智齿发炎、口腔溃疡、脂溢性脱发、痤疮、便秘、淋巴结节、月经不调、不孕不育、泌尿生殖系统感染、过敏性疾病等。

少阴性颠倒反常，区块最为狭隘却又能宏越水火二性。少阴的原始本质就是伏邪托透的枢机，也是促阴证化阳证最关键的时期，所以在《伤寒论》三阴篇中唯少阴篇幅最大。我们也可以这样理解，少阴病可以是普通慢性病转为阴性危重症与沉疴痼疾的过渡期，后世出于对称化、系统化和为了便于理解，将其假托为阴性表证。

exterior-interior, upper-lower and yin-yang because of its wide range of diseases and blurred boundaries. As a result, the Shaoyang likes clear and freedom but hates depression and stagnation. The corresponding physiological age group from Yangming to Shaoyang mainly focuses on young adults, during which the gradual coordination between rationality and sensibility caused by withdrawal of Yang and release of Yin. The body will not only cater to the liberation and spreading of Shaoyang, but also adapt to the rhythm of soul growth and maturity. Otherwise, it will generate the frenetic stirring or depression and stagnation of ministerial fire, causing autonomic nerve disorder, anxiety neurosis, hyperthyroidism, alimentary canal ulcers, cholecystitis, myocarditis, pulmonary tuberculosis, nasopharyngitis, wisdom tooth inflammation, mouth ulcer, alopecia seborrheica, acne, constipation, lymphoid nodules, irregular menses, infertility, genitourinary system infection, allergic diseases, etc.

Shaoyin is in a topsy-turvy nature, and its area is the narrowest but can control both sides of fire and water in human body. The original essence of Shaoyin is a pivot to expel latent pathogen, and it is also the most critical period to promote Yin syndrome into Yang syndrome. Therefore, in the triple-yin disease of *Shanghan Lun*, only Shaoyin has the largest length. We can also understand that Shaoyin disease can be the transition period from common chronic

基于少阴病的特质，我们可以及早在少阴枢机上做干预治疗与截断以防止患者内陷太阴和厥阴，这也是本概述讨论研究癌前病变的核心落脚点。从少阳至少阴对应的生理年龄段主要集中在中青年时期和中老年初期，此期间也是诸多癌前病变的病理聚合矛盾凸显最频繁的时期，也是诸如高血压、心脏病、糖尿病、慢性肝炎等慢性大病的暴发期。现代临床医学统计数据曾明确指出：无论男女，当超过55岁后，癌症的发病率就开始呈指数性地上升。这也进一步印证与回扣了我们所做出的结论，毫无疑问，少阴病理期是现代人群濒临患癌的指数爆炸的起点。

具体到中医药在少阴区块的免疫介入方面，笔者尝试引用免疫学的相关基础概念做出以下阐释：

免疫细胞中的T淋巴细胞成熟于"心系"，即西医所谓的胸腺——一个位于胸部正中，心脏上方的功能组织，

disease to critical and difficult Yin disease. And for the sake of symmetry, systematization and easy understanding, the later generations refer to it as the exterior pattern of Yin.

Based on the characteristics of Shaoyin disease, we can intervene on Shaoyin pivot as early as possible to prevent patients from getting worse into Taiyin and Jueyin disease, which is also the core foothold of the study of precancerous lesions in this outline. The corresponding physiological age group from Shaoyang to Shaoyin mainly focuses on the young and middle age, which is the most frequent period of the concentration of pathological contradictions of many precancerous lesions, and is also the explosive stage of chronic serious diseases such as hypertension, heart disease, diabetes and chronic hepatitis. The modern clinical statistics have made it clear that the incidence of cancer begins to rise exponentially when it comes to men and women over the age of 55, which further confirms our conclusion. There is no doubt that Shaoyin pathological period is the starting point of index explosion on the verge of cancer for modern population.

In terms of the immune intervention of TCM in Shaoyin pivot, the author tries to quote the relevant basic concepts of immunology to make the following explanation:

The T lymphocytes are the functional basis of Shaoyin's "protection in the surface of human body", the so-called "backup club" of cellular immunity. And they mature in

这是少阴"心部于表"的功能基础,即所谓的细胞免疫的"后援会"。免疫B细胞则成熟于骨髓,得肾精之濡养,这是少阴"肾治于里"的功能基础,负责抗体的产生与介导体液免疫应答。T细胞和B细胞都来源于造血干细胞,这种生命的原始物质与我们中医理论中的"真阳元气"有着深刻的交集。当胸腺功能紊乱或功能降低时,B细胞因失去T细胞的控制而功能亢进,就可能产生大量自身抗体,并引起各种自身免疫病。同样,在某些情况下,B细胞也可控制或增强T细胞的功能。由此可见,身体中各类免疫反应,不论是细胞免疫还是体液免疫,共同构成了一个极为精细、复杂而完善的防卫体系。我们中医整体辨证论治的优势也于此彰显无遗。所以笔者自始至终认为,少阴病在当今临床中的延展力是无穷大的。

太阴是机体后天生、运、化、动的基础和根本,任何生命活动的能量精微都来源于它。也可以这样讲,太阴充

the "heart system" in TCM theory, the so-called thymus in modern medicine — A functional tissue located in the middle of the chest and above the heart. The B lymphocytes are the functional basis of Shaoyin's "protection inside of the human body", which mature in bone marrow and nourished by kidney essence, and they are also responsible for the production of antibody and mediate humoral immune response. The T lymphocytes and B lymphocytes come from hematopoietic stem cells which are the primitive substance of life and have a profound intersection with "primordial Yang" in TCM theory. When the thymic function is disordered or decreased, the B lymphocytes are hyperfunctional due to the loss of T lymphocytes' control. It may produce a large number of autoantibodies and cause a variety of autoimmune diseases. Similarly, the B lymphocytes can control or enhance the function of T lymphocytes in some cases. Thus it can be seen that all kinds of immune responses in the body, whether cellular or humoral immunity, together constitute a very fine, complex and perfect defense system. The advantages of syndrome differentiation and treatment of holistic view of TCM are also obvious here. Therefore, the author believes from beginning to end that the extensibility of Shaoyin disease in today's clinic is infinite.

Taiyin is the foundation of the generation, promotion, transformation and movement of the body's acquired

满了坤土色彩,在整个生命系统中扮演了"地母盖亚"的角色。同时太阴区块是人类潜意识与内心世界的"存储卡",因此也容易富集诸多精神和肉体的暗能量。从少阴至太阴对应的生理年龄段主要集中在中老年和老年时期,在此期间诸多腑气衰败导致的疑难病症亦伴随有明显的高发趋势,如消化道功能性梗阻、消化道恶性肿瘤等,同时诸多太阴风寒湿表证引起的痹证、痿证等以及太阴浊阴上犯引起的痴呆、郁证、脑血管疾病等亦可常见于临床。

厥阴乃"两阴交尽",是生命发展的最后一个能量级。本身是一种阴阳否格的表现——肝阴耗竭,肾阳离绝,阴阳各失其守,呈逆乱崩绝之象。生死关头在厥阴病里往往呈现极端化的表现,作为医生真正把握起来难免力不从心,临床的受挫感也很强。因为多数的厥阴病已经出现了毒邪泛滥成巢的局面,类似于千疮百孔的"蜂窝煤",与

constitution, and the essence of energy in any life activity is derived from it. It can also be said that the Taiyin is full of the kun-earth temperament, and it plays the role of the "earth mother Gaia" throughout the life system. In addition, Taiyin is the "memory card" of the human subconsciousness and the inner world, so it is easy to concentrate plenty of dark energy of spirit and body. The corresponding physiological age group from Shaoyin to Taiyin mainly focuses on the elderly age, during which the complicated and difficult diseases caused by the exhaustion of Qi in the Fu-organs such as the functional obstruction and malignant tumor of the digestive tract also have a marked high-incidence tendency. At the same time, plenty of the arthralgia, atrophy-flaccidity, etc. caused by the Taiyin's wind-cold-damp exterior syndrome, and the dementia, depression syndrome, cerebrovascular disease, etc. caused by the harassment of Taiyin's turbid Yin are also common in the clinic.

Jueyin is the mergence of double Yin and is the last energy level of the development of life. It is a kind of expression of partition of Yin and Yang — The exhaustion of liver Yin and kidney Yang leads to Yin and Yang losing control of each other, which shows the ending of chaos and annihilation. It is shown that there is often extreme appearance in Jueyin disease at the moment of life and death. It is inevitable for a doctor to deal with them under a severe sense

之相伴随的便是正气的耗损至极,笔者将其称为"厥阴堕落型稳态",整体呈"变态性"推进,甚则最终导致《黄帝内经》与《伤寒论》中"死,不治"的结局。从太阴至厥阴对应的生理年龄段主要集中在老年和暮年时期,在此期间诸多脏气衰败导致的疑难病症亦伴随有明显的高发趋势,如肺癌、肝癌、胰腺癌、心肾衰竭等。

众所周知,恶性肿瘤的本质是一类细胞生长周期异常的疾病。笔者认为,细胞周期功能异常亦即阴盛阳衰的微观表现。阳衰可以看作细胞周期功能失调与人体免疫功能失常;阴盛可以看作细胞的无限增殖与恶性肿瘤的免疫逃避。《黄帝内经》有云:"阳气者,烦劳则张",过度烦劳会导致阳衰而阴张;"凡阴阳之要,阳密乃固",阳不密则阴阳不固;"阳气者,若天与日,失其所则折寿而不彰,故天运当以日光明",高度评价了阳气对于机体寿命与生命质量彰显的核心调控作用,文中的"天运当以日光明"

of clinical frustration. Most of the Jueyin diseases have already formed a situation where pathogenic toxins detain stubbornly into "nests" similar to the "honeycomb coal" full of holes, which is accompanied by the extreme loss of healthy Qi. The author calls this kind of situation the "degenerate steady state of Jueyin". The whole process is deteriorating, even leading to the ending of incurables recorded in *Huangdi Neijing* and *Shanghan Lun*. The corresponding physiological age group from Taiyin to Jueyin mainly focuses on the declining age, during which the complicated and difficult diseases caused by the exhaustion of Qi in the Zang-organs such as lung cancer, liver cancer, pancreatic cancer, heart failure and kidney failure also have a marked high-incidence tendency.

It is well known that the essence of malignant tumor is a kind of disease with abnormal cell growth cycle. The author believes that abnormal cell cycle function is the microscopic manifestation of Yin exuberance with Yang debilitation. The Yang debilitation can be regarded as cell cycle and immune dysfunction; the Yin exuberance can be regarded as the infinite proliferation of cells and the immune escape of malignant tumors. As *Huangdi Neijing* contained: "Overstrain will make Yang Qi overdrawn", excessive anxiety and fatigue will finally lead to Yin exuberance with Yang debilitation; "The essential principle in all interactions of Yin and Yang is to have the Yang sealed in the body, and thereby, to ensure its firmness", if

则明确指出人体生命活动正常而有序的运作机制离不了阳气的温煦与统摄功能。由此我们可以看出阳气在恶性肿瘤防治中的重要作用。

the Yang is not sealed in the body, it will lead to the partition of Yin and Yang; "Yang Qi is just like the sun in the sky, it's abnormal flow shortens people's life and reduces quality of life, thus the normal movement of the heavens depends on the normal luminosity of the sun", which highly evaluates the core readjustment and controlling effect of Yang Qi on the span and quality of life. The "normal movement of the heavens depends on the normal luminosity of the sun" explained above makes it clear that the normal and orderly operation mechanism of life depends on the function of Yang Qi. Therefore, we can see the important role of Yang Qi in the prevention and treatment of malignant tumors.

八、中医辨证观下癌前病变治法的探讨

"温补太阴,托透少阴,清宣少阳"是癌前病变的核心治法。

综合《伤寒论》六经辨证的整体观,我们可以比较系统地窥探到:针对癌前病变人群,只要把患者本身所禀赋的不同的太阴能量阈值加以提高,进而带动患者自身不同维度少阴枢机的生运化动,患者自身病理超稳态结构多样的病理基质就可以经由少阳三焦畅达通泄,从而使患者恢复到与个体生理阶段相一致的"阴平阳秘"的理想体质状态。这便是我们中药免疫疗法癌前介入的核心突破点,我们也由此确立了"温补太阴,托透少阴,清宣少阳"的系统治疗原则。

笔者认为,由《伤寒论》六经辨证确立的"温补太

VIII. Discussion on the Treatment of Precancerous Lesions under the View of Syndrome Differentiation in TCM

Warming and supplementing Taiyin, drawing and expelling through Shaoyin, and clearing in Shaoyang are the core treatments of precancerous lesions.

Referring to the holistic view of the six-meridian syndrome differentiation in *Shanghan Lun*, we can peek into more systematically that as for the people with precancerous lesions, as long as the different Taiyin's energy threshold value of the patient is increased, and then the generation, promotion, transformation and movement of Shaoyin pivot of different dimensions of the patient is put in motion, causing the diverse pathological substrates of the patient's pathological hyper-stable structure can be expelled unobstructedly via the triple energizer membrane of Shaoyang, so that the patient can be restored to the ideal constitution state of "Yin and Yang are balanced and sealed" which is consistent with the individual physiological phase. That is the core breakthrough point of the precancerous intervention of TCM immunotherapy, and from this we have established the principle of systematic treatments of "warming and supplementing Taiyin, drawing and expelling through Shaoyin, and clearing in Shaoyang".

The author believes that the treatments of "warming

阴，托透少阴，清宣少阳"的治法是《黄帝内经》反治法的极致发挥，也是癌前病变这类潜隐能力强、持续时间长、病理稳态明显、病理机制复杂、危害性大且具有逆转可能性的慢性疑难病症的最佳切入点。著名伤寒学者娄绍昆先生也同样认为："反治法的适应证是某些复杂的、顽固的、用正治法虽然辨证无误却治疗无效的疾病。这类疾病往往是一些可逆性的慢性病。它的复杂性表现在临床可见寒热兼夹、虚实错杂、病象丛生。它的顽固性表现在正气受挫，邪毒胶着不去阻滞气机，形成痰、瘀等病理代谢产物。"

and supplementing Taiyin, drawing and expelling through Shaoyin, and clearing in Shaoyang" which established by the six-meridian syndrome differentiation in *Shanghan Lun* are the ultimate play of the paradoxical treatment in *Huangdi Neijing*, and are also the best entry points for chronic and difficult diseases such as precancerous lesions which have strong latent ability, long duration, obvious pathological homeostasis, complex pathological mechanism, great harmfulness and the possibility of reversal. Lou Shaokun also thinks that "The indications of the paradoxical treatment are some complex and stubborn diseases which are treated by explicable treatment under the correct syndrome differentiation but of no avail. These type of diseases are usually some reversible chronic diseases. Their complexities in the clinical may be represented as multiple morbidity of the intermingled cold-heat and deficiency-excess. Their refractory natures mainly manifest in the pathogenic poison detaining stubbornly and obstructing the movement of Qi caused by the frustration of healthy Qi, resulting in the formation of pathological metabolic products such as dampness turbidity and accumulated stasis in the end."

九、中药免疫疗法癌前介入的基本原则与代表方剂

【基本原则】

1. 立足伤寒六经钤法,排除非特异性干扰。亦即《黄帝内经》所云:"知标与本,用之不殆,明知逆顺,正行无问,此之谓也。"

2. 明确瞑眩反应本质(定义、机制与作用),排除临床药源性疾病的干扰。

3. 治疗期间充分利用好现代医学诊断,及时排查治疗过程中非医疗因素下患者自身的疾病隐患,避免临床小概率事件的发生。(主要集中在急性心脑血管疾病与急腹症,如急性心肌梗死、动脉瘤、急性胰腺炎等,此时西医的及时介入支持治疗尤为重要。)

4. 建立并完善相关病房制度,排除时间、空间、医疗条件的局限性。

IX. The Basic Principles and Representative Formulas of Precancerous Intervention in Immunotherapy of TCM

【 Basic Principles 】

1. Be based on the six-meridian syndrome differentiation of *Shanghan Lun* and eliminate the non-specific interferences. Exactly as emphasized in *Huangdi Neijing*: "Awareness of branch and root ensures successful treatment, and understanding the methods of contrary therapy and conforming therapy guarantees correct treatment."

2. Clear the nature of dizziness reaction (definition, mechanism and function) and eliminate the interferences of clinical drug-induced diseases.

3. Make full use of the modern medical diagnosis during the treatment to check the hidden danger without medical sake of patient's own disease in time in order to avoid the occurrence of the clinical small-probability events which are mainly focused on acute cardiovascular and cerebrovascular diseases such as acute myocardial infarction and aneurysm and acute abdominal diseases such as acute pancreatitis. At this time, the timely intervention support of modern medicine is especially important.

4. Establish and improve the relevant ward system, and overcome the limitation of time, space and medical condition.

5. 治疗对象建议控制在 55 岁以下，无慢性大病基础病史。

【代表方剂】

①九鼎归宗饮

②天一饮

【方剂组成】

①九鼎归宗饮：

肉桂 15～45g，赤芍 15～45g，柴胡 15～45g，生半夏 15～45g，苍术 15～45g，茯苓 20～60g，干姜 15～45g，生附子 15～45g，生甘草 10～30g，大枣 20～60g。

②天一饮：

茯苓 20～60g，肉桂 15～45g，生半夏 15～45g，干姜 15～45g，生附子 15～45g，生甘草 10～30g。

5. It is recommended that the treatment object should be controlled under the age of 55 without the basic history of chronic serious diseases.

【 Representative Formulas 】

① Jiuding Guizong Decoction

② Tian-yi Decoction

【 Composition of Decoction 】

① Jiuding Guizong Decoction:

Cortex Cinnamomi 15~45g; Radix Paeoniae Rubra 15~45g; Radix Bupleuri 15~45g; Raw Pinellia Tuber 15~45g; Rhizoma Atractylodis 15~45g; Poria 20~60g; Dried Ginger 15~45g; Raw Radix Aconiti Lateralis Preparata 15~45g; Raw Radix Glycyrrhizae 10~30g; Fructus Jujubae 20~60g.

② Tian-yi Decoction:

Poria 20~60g; Cortex Cinnamomi 15~45g; Raw Pinellia Tuber 15~45g; Dried Ginger 15~45g; Raw Radix Aconiti Lateralis Preparata 15~45g; Raw Radix Glycyrrhizae 10~30g.

十、九鼎归宗饮加减与服药须知

【九鼎归宗饮加减】

1. 倘若患者出现：白天易嗜睡低迷、体重明显超重、汗出小便异常、患有顽固性皮肤病并未得到彻底根治、关节肌肉疼痛怕冷、凌晨三到五点钟易醒、缓慢性心律失常、素有肺系疾病中任意三种或三种以上情况（麻黄三联征），酌加麻黄 10～30g、杏仁 10～30g。

2. 倘若患者出现：舌下或舌两侧瘀络瘀点明显、身体部位异常刺痛、双侧腹股沟附近明显压痛甚则伴有抵抗感中任意一种或一种以上情况，酌加桃仁 10～30g。

3. 倘若患者出现胸腹部胀闷不适，如有气聚抟结不散之感，酌加厚朴 15～45g；如若伴有明显胀痛感，酌加枳壳 15～45g。

X. Variations of Jiuding Guizong Decoction and Instructions for Taking Medicine

【 Variations of Jiuding Guizong Decoction 】

1. 10~30g of Raw Ephedra and Semen Armeniacau Amarum are added as appropriate if the patient shows any three or more of the following conditions (the triple sign of Ephedra):

Feeling drowsy and listless during the day; Being overweight; Having abnormal sweat and urination; Having intractable dermatosis that has not been completely cured; Having cold pain in joints and muscles; Waking up from 03:00 to 05:00 frequently; Having Bradyarrhythmia; Suffering from disease of respiratory system.

2. 10~30g of Semen Persicae is added as appropriate if the patient shows any one or more of the following conditions:

Having obvious blood stasis collaterals or points under or on the side of the tongue; Having abnormal tingling at parts of the body; Having obvious tenderness and even the sense of resistance around the bilateral groins.

3. 15~45g of Cortex Magnoliae Officinalis is added as appropriate if the patient shows the discomfort of thoracic or abdominal distention such as having a sense of gas gathering without dissipating, and 15~45g of Fructus Aurantii is added as appropriate if the patient is accompanied by obvious distending pain.

4. 倘若患者出现：形体羸瘦、营养不良、食欲不振、心下痞闷、气力不足、二便及汗出异常而致阴液耗损较明显中任意两种或两种以上的情况，酌加人参 10～30g、怀山药 30～90g。

注：以上配药在患者治疗期间出现明显改善后即可去掉。

【服药须知】

1. 九鼎归宗饮、天一饮隔天交替服用；

2. 早上九点、下午三点、晚上九点各一次，加热温服；

3. 忌口生、冷、水果；

4. 治疗期间停用西药，如有依赖性可呈阶梯式逐渐停药；

5. 妇女经期不停药；

6. 建议配合长期艾灸，膻中、中脘、关元与内关、足三里、三阴交两组配穴隔天交替艾灸。

4. 10~30g of Radix Ginseng and 30~90g of Rhizoma Dioscoreae are added as appropriate if the patient shows any two or more of the following conditions:

Being thin and weak; Being malnourished; Having poor appetite; Suffering the discomfort of epigastric stuffiness; Feeling hypodynamic; Having obvious loss of body fluids caused by abnormal urination, defecation and sweating.

Note: The variations explained above can be removed after significant improvement during treatment.

【 Instructions for Taking Medicine 】

1. The Jiuding Guizong Decoction and Tian-yi Decoction should be taken alternately every other day;

2. The medicine needs to be taken altogether 3 times while it is warm at 9: 00 in the morning, 3: 00 in the afternoon and 9: 00 in the evening every day;

3. Ban eating raw food, cold food and fruit;

4. Stop taking western medicine during treatment. If the patient is dependent on it, the western medicine could be stopped step by step;

5. Women should not stop taking Chinese medicine during the menstruation;

6. It is suggested to cooperate with moxibustion during treatment, the two sets of points (① Tanzhong, Zhongwan and Guanyuan; ② Neiguan, Zusanli and Sanyinjiao) can be taken alternately every other day.

十一、中药免疫疗法癌前介入的治疗转归

1. 免疫初期

大多集中在患者开始正式接受治疗 3～6 个月内,此期间患者如若出现比较轻微的反应,可以守方不变。也有极少数患者在治疗初期即可发生由免疫初期到免疫抑制期转变的全过程,说明患者自身免疫应答与代偿能力较为灵敏,自身病理稳态程度较轻,遇到这种情况发生时仅需按照治疗转归的基本治疗原则处理即可。

2. 免疫激期

大多集中在患者开始正式接受治疗 3～6 个月后,此期间患者易发生"倒带式反应",即依靠人体自身强大的生理记忆能力,患者会多次重复出现之前曾患疾病的些许症状,可以撤去天一饮。

XI. Treatment Stages of Precancerous Intervention in Immunotherapy of TCM

1. Initial Stage of Immunization

The initial stage of immunization is mainly within 3~6 months after the patients began to receive the treatment. During this stage, the decoction can be remained unchanged if the patients have slight reactions. There are also very few patients who can change wholly from initial stage of immunization to immunosuppressive stage in the early stage of treatment, which indicates that the autoimmune response and compensation ability of the patients are more sensitive, and the degree of homeostasis of their own pathology is relatively lesser. We can deal with this situation according to the basic principles of treatment stages.

2. Intensification Stage of Immunization

The intensification stage of immunization is mainly after when the patients have received the treatment for about 3~6 months. During this stage, the patients are prone to arise "rewind reaction" relying on the body's own strong physical memory ability, and then the patients will repeatedly appear some symptoms of the previous diseases many times. At this moment, the Tian-yi Decoction can be removed.

3. 免疫调平期

免疫激期过后，注意在患者续服九鼎归宗饮的基础上密切观察，当患者出现典型且比较剧烈的瞑眩反应后，随即可以出现两种不同的转归：对于三阴体质患者，整体反应基本不会过渡到免疫抑制期，此时在继续服用九鼎归宗饮的基础上结合相对应的瞑眩反应基本处理原则继续治疗即可；对于少阳内陷三阴体质者，整体反应基本会向免疫抑制期过渡，且比较剧烈，具体情况参下。

4. 免疫抑制期

对于少阳内陷三阴体质者，患者的瞑眩反应会比较明显，主要集中于皮肤、呼吸系统、消化系统和泌尿生殖系统的急性炎症，此时将九鼎归宗饮中的附子去掉：

倘若患者出现口干口渴明显、高热不退，酌加生石膏 $30 \sim 90g$、知母 $15 \sim 45g$，伴有不汗出或喘者，酌加麻黄 $10 \sim 30g$、杏仁 $10 \sim 30g$；

3. Leveling Stage of Immunization

After the intensification stage of immunization, it is essential to closely observe the patients continuing taking Jiuding Guizong Decoction. When the typical and intense dizziness reaction appears, there can be two different outcomes: For patients with triple-yin constitution, the overall reaction will not transition to the immunosuppressive stage in general. At this time, the treatment can be continued referring to the corresponding basic treatment principle of the dizziness reaction on the basis of continuing taking the Jiuding Guizong Decoction; For the patients with constitution that Shaoyang invades triple-yin, the more intense overall reaction will transition to the immunosuppressive stage in general. For details, please refer to the following.

4. Immunosuppressive Stage

For the patients with constitution that Shaoyang invades triple-yin, the dizziness reaction will be obvious and mainly focus on the acute inflammation of the skin, respiratory system, digestive system and genitourinary system. At this time, the Raw Radix Aconiti Lateralis Preparata in Jiuding Guizong Decoction can be removed:

30~90g of Gypsum Fibrosum and 15~45g of Rhizoma Anemarrhenae are added as appropriate if the patient feels dry and thirsty obviously in the mouth and has non-return high fever, and 10~30g of Raw Ephedra and Semen

倘若患者出现胸内烦闷扰乱、身体孔窍部位上火、皮肤遍布痘疹、胃内嘈杂上逆反酸并伴有口苦、舌苔变厚变腻变干或变黄、身目发黄、总胆红素和转氨酶升高，酌加生栀子15～45g、豆豉15～45g，实热或郁热偏重者酌加黄芩10～45g、黄连5～30g；

倘若患者出现大小便不通利、腹部硬满疼痛甚则可触及肿物而拒按，酌加生大黄5～30g、芒硝5～15g，里实严重且来势猛烈者（伴有腹膜刺激征），酌加甘遂1～5g。

值得注意的是，极少数患者会因为中药免疫疗法激活人体的生理对抗系统、动摇机体的病理稳态而致使患者潜

Armeniacau Amarum are added as appropriate if the patient is accompanied by a non-sweating or dyspnea;

15~45g of Raw Fructus Gardeniae and 15~45g of Semen Sojae Preparatum are added as appropriate if the patient has the dysphoria and harass in the chest, discomforts related to "the fire characterized by flaring up" such as inflammation occurring frequently in the orifices of the body, skin covered with rash, gastric noise and acid regurgitation accompanied by a sense of bitter in the mouth, tongue coating becoming thicker, greasier, drier or yellower, yellow skin and eyes, or elevated total bilirubin and transaminase, and 10~45g of Radix Scutellariae and 5~30g Rhizoma Coptidis are added as appropriate if the excess or stagnated heat of the patient is serious;

5~30g of Raw Radix et Rhizoma Rhei and 5~15g of Natrii Sulfas are added as appropriate if the patient has the difficulty in urination and defecation or abdominal hardness and fullness with pain which even is accompanied by palpable mass and resistance after palpation, and 1~5g of Radix Euphorbiae Kansui is added as appropriate if the interior excess of the patient is severe and violent (Accompanied by peritoneal irritation sign).

It is worth noting that very few patients will be led to the early appearance of potential early malignant tumors such as carcinoma in situ because the TCM immunotherapy can

在的诸如原位癌等早期恶性肿瘤提前出现。与常规恶性肿瘤患者不同，这些患者大多都会在恶性肿瘤提前产生的初期即出现身体上的明显不适，这也提示了在治疗期间现代医学的针对性检查及时介入的重要性。早期癌症一经及时发现与确认，为避免延误患者病情，医生应当遵从"标而本之"的临床诊治思路，适当结合现代肿瘤外科切除术及时清除原发灶，术后经络受损与术后后遗症则应优先选用中药进行治疗。

5. 免疫恢复期

当三阴体质患者的免疫调平期与少阳内陷三阴体质患者的免疫抑制期度过后，可以撤去九鼎归宗饮加减方。恢复期治疗主张从脾阴立法，根据李东垣"阳旺则能生阴血"的理论，同时为避免贼邪死灰复燃之势，处以桂枝汤补虚加味方：

activate the physiological antagonistic system and shake the pathological homeostasis of the human body. Different from the conventional patients with malignant tumors, most of these patients will have obvious physical discomforts in the stage of the early generation of malignant tumors, which also suggests the importance of timely intervention in the targeted examination of modern medicine during the treatment. Once the early cancer is detected and confirmed in time, in order to avoid delaying the patient's condition, the doctors should abide by the clinical thinking of "First treat its tip and afterwards treat its root" in *Huangdi Neijing* and properly make use of the modern tumor surgery to clear up the primary tumor in time, and the damages of meridians and the sequelae after operation should be treated with traditional Chinese medicine as a priority.

5. Recovery Stage of Immunization

When the leveling stage of immunization of the patients with triple-yin constitution and the immunosuppressive stage of the patients with constitution that Shaoyang invades triple-yin have passed, the modified formula of Jiuding Guizong Decoction can be removed. The author advocates the enlightenment from spleen Yin in the course of recovery treatment according to Li Dongyuan's theory that "The production of Yin-blood depends on the exuberance of spleen Yang". And in order to avoid the resurgence of pathogen

肉桂 15～45g，白芍 15～45g，生姜 15～45g，大枣 20～60g，生甘草 10～30g，人参 10～30g，怀山药 30～90g。

饮食上可摄取适量烂牛蹄与猪蹄筋、白花胶、小米山药南瓜粥、山药汁、当归生姜羊肉汤等，忌口生、冷、水果。

like thief, the supplemented Cortex Cinnamomi Tonifying Decoction is recommended:

Cortex Cinnamomi 15~45g; Radix Paeoniae Alba 15~45g; Fresh Ginger 15~45g; Fructus Jujubae 20~60g; Raw Radix Glycyrrhizae 10~30g; Radix Ginseng 10~30g; Rhizoma Dioscoreae 30~90g.

A proper amount of stewed cattle and pig tendon; swim bladder of the culter alburnus; millet, yam and pumpkin porridge; Rhizoma Dioscoreae juice; Tangkuei, Fresh Ginger and Mutton Decoction; etc. can be taken up on the diet, but the raw food, cold food and fruit are prohibited.

十二、中药免疫疗法癌前介入的瞑眩反应及其基本处理原则

1.舌头、脸及四肢发麻或出现过电感。一般主要集中发生在服药初期,是药物搜刮经络的表现,患者多为经络敏感体质,此情况一般不做处理,不适感可在短期内自行消失。需要注意的是,倘若患者相继伴随头晕目眩或眼前发黑时,务必确保患者及时卧床休息,以免因摔倒而发生意外。

2.颈肩腰背部僵凝酸痛,关节肌肉疼痛或怕冷。出现此类表现的患者一般有三种情况:既往患有风寒湿痹证,或患有慢性肺系疾病,或曾经出现过经络损伤。治疗期间会出现药物修复过程与托邪外出的连锁反应。基本处理原则为先予局部拔罐后局部外涂药酒覆被保鲜膜配合局部热敷或温灸,继用针刺松解术,以经筋刺法(阳陵泉为主穴,局部阿是为配穴)与五输穴(输主体重节痛)取穴为主。每日1次,10天为1疗程,常规情况下1~2疗程即可明显改善。

XII. Dizziness Reactions and Their Basic Treatment Principles of Precancerous Intervention in Immunotherapy of TCM

1. The patient might have a sense of numbness or electric on the tongue, face and limbs. This kind of sense is mainly concentrated in the early stage of taking decoction, and it is the manifestation of the decoction clearing the meridians. And the patient is likely to have the meridian-sensitive constitution. This situation generally does not need to be dealt with, and the discomfort can disappear in the short term. It should be noted that if the patient has been accompanied by dizziness or darkness of vision, be sure to ensure that the patient stays in bed in time to avoid accidents due to falls.

2. The patient might have discomforts at shoulder, neck and back and cold pains at joints and muscles. There are generally three cases of patients in such circumstances that the patients previously suffered from arthralgia of wind-cold-damp, chronic respiratory system disease or meridian injury, which leads to the chain reactions of repair and detox of the decoction during the treatment. The basic treatment principles are to cup the affected part first, then apply the medicinal wine covered with the fresh-keeping film to the affected part and cooperate with the hot compress or moxibustion at the same time, and then use the channel sinew acupuncture technique

附 药酒方：麻黄15g，肉桂15g，生附子15g，苍术15g，生姜30g，以50度白酒没过药物浸泡5天即可使用。（仅限于外用，严禁内服）

3. 烦躁不安，频繁上火，以身体孔窍部位为主（眼、耳、鼻、口、咽喉、二阴）。出现此类表现的患者大部分既往长期情志不遂。中医理论认为人体五脏、五志与人体机窍相互连属感召，长期郁滞的不良情绪郁而化火可以加快人体的癌变进程。治疗期间患者过往的怫郁五志可以通过机窍出现"火郁发之"的表现。基本处理原则为宣通郁结、透热转气，酌加生栀子15～45g、豆豉15～45g。

(Take Yanglingquan as the main point and the Ashi as the supporting point) and the loosening method which is mainly based on taking the acupoints of the five transport points (The transport point can treat pain in the joints of the body). The patients should be treated 10 days as a course once a day, and the dizziness reaction could be significantly relieved after 1~2 courses of treatment in general.

Appendix

Composition of the medicinal wine (External use, prohibit internal use):

Raw Ephedra 15g; Cortex Cinnamomi 15g; Raw Radix Aconiti Lateralis Preparata 15g; Rhizoma Atractylodis 15g; Fresh Ginger 30g.

Soak the above medicinal herbs with about 500mL of liquor (50% vol) for 5 days.

3. The patient might have dysphoria and discomforts related to "the fire characterized by flaring up" such as inflammation occurring frequently mainly in the orifices of the body (eye, ear, nose, mouth, throat, anus and external genitalia). Most of the patients with this kind of manifestation have long term affect-mind dissatisfaction. The TCM theory holds that the five Zang-organs, the five emotions and the orifices of the human body are interrelated and inductive with each other, and the bad mood of long-term depression can transform into fire which can speed up the process of

4.面部、四肢出现浮肿，小便不易排出。这是治疗期间人体湿邪引动外溢三焦膜腠的表现。基本处理原则为通利水道、去菀陈莝，可针刺双侧阴陵泉（沿太阴脾经循行逆方向呈30°进针1.5～2寸）、双侧三阴交（沿胫骨内侧缘呈45°进针1～1.5寸）、双侧委阳，施以中幅度提插手法15～30秒，以出现麻电放射感为度，每日1次，10天为1疗程，常规情况下1～2疗程即可明显改善。另水肿而喘者，酌加麻黄10～30g、杏仁10～30g，水邪泛滥三焦甚则出现典型体腔积液（以胸腔、心包、腹腔积液较为常见）表现酌加甘遂1～5g。

carcinogenesis. During the treatment, the patients' past depressed emotions can be expressed through the "dispersion of stagnant fire" of the orifices. And the basic treatment principle is to clear the depression, stagnation and heat from Ying-fen to Qi-fen through taking 15~45g of Raw Fructus Gardeniae and 15~45g of Semen Sojae Preparatum as appropriate.

4. The patient might have edema in the face and limbs and inhibited urination. This is the expression of triple energizer membrane caused by dampness pathogen in human body during the treatment. And the basic treatment principles are to free the waterways and remove the long-standing dregs in the body — Acupuncture can be done on both sides of Yinlingquan (Enter the needle 1.5~2 inches at 30° against the direction of the spleen meridian), Sanyinjiao (Enter the needle 1~1.5 inches at 45° along the medial edge of the tibia) and Weiyang with 15~30 seconds of medium-amplitude lifting-thrusting method based on the aim of the occurrence of radiosensitivity. The patients should be treated 10 days as a course once a day, and the dizziness reaction could be significantly relieved after 1~2 courses of treatment in general. It is worth emphasizing that 10~30g of Raw Ephedra and Semen Armeniacau Amarum could be added as appropriate if the patients have dyspnea and edema, and 1~5g of Radix Euphorbiae Kansui could be added as appropriate if there are

5.全身出现淤斑、丘疹、痘疮或溃疡,尤以头面部、四肢为主,少数患者亦会出现在生殖区附近,会伴有不同程度的痛痒感,局部主要表现为红肿热痛。若患者素有皮肤病、关节炎、痛风等表位疾病,这些疾病短期内可能会出现加重。中医经典《黄帝内经》里曾强调过:"善治者治皮毛,其次治肌肤,其次治筋脉,其次治六腑,其次治五脏。治五脏者,半死半生也。"中医理论认为,久病可由经络传至脏腑,中药免疫治疗的核心便是扶助正气、托透邪气,患者在治疗期间自身机体开始出现正邪交争的层层递进,进而导致邪气逐渐由脏腑传至其相对应经络,最终以人体表位的急性炎症为主要矛盾凸显与透发渠道,完成对疾病消除的动态转化与阴阳调平。基本处理原则为外用鬼门消解方泡酒或浸油擦拭患处,服完中药后用热水泡脚发汗(足胫处有溃疡者除外,要求水位没过三阴交),针刺八风、八邪,对太阳穴、后背督脉及膀胱经侧线、曲池、阳陵泉、血海、委中及起疹子的部位刺络拔罐放血,风池予以刮痧,以局部紫红为度。部分病理稳态较重、疾

body cavity effusions (Hydrothorax, hydropericardium and ascites are more common in clinic) caused by the overflow of dampness pathogen in triple energizer membrane.

5. The patient might have ecchymosis, pox rash or ulcer with different degree of pain, itch and regional manifestations of redness, swelling or hot pain on the whole body (Obvious on head, face and limbs, a few will also appear on the genital area). If the patients have already suffered from exterior syndromes such as skin diseases, arthritis and gout, these kinds of diseases may be exacerbated in short term during the treatment. It has been emphasized in *Huangdi Neijing* that "Excellent doctors treat diseases when pathogenic factors have just invaded the skin; ordinary doctors treat diseases when pathogenic factors have deepened into the muscles...Once the five Zang-organs are involved, the disease is fatal". According to the TCM theory, the long-term disease can be transmitted from meridians to Zang-fu organs. The core of TCM immunotherapy is to help the healthy Qi fight against and dispel the pathogenic Qi. During the treatment, the patients themselves begin to show the progressive situation of the struggle between healthy and pathogenic Qi, which leads to the gradual transmission of pathogenic Qi from the Zang-fu organs to their corresponding meridians, and finally takes the acute inflammation of human body exterior as the main contradiction and detoxification channel to complete

病潜伏较深的患者反应时间可长达数月，此时应予以患者一定的精神鼓励与耐心解释，以增强患者的信心与理解。

附 鬼门消解方：黄芩、黄连、生大黄、生栀子、苍术、茯苓、生甘草、桃仁、赤芍、芒硝等份适量，切碎或研末，浸入50度白酒或纯芝麻油中5天即可外用。（仅限于外用，严禁内服）

the dynamic transformation of disease elimination and the yin-yang balance. The basic treatment principles are to scrub the affected area with Guimen Xiaojie Formula, sweat through soaking feet in hot water after taking the decoction (Except for patients with ulcers on the feet and tibia, and the required water level of the hot water should be higher than the point of Sanyinjiao), take the acupuncture at Bafeng and Baxie points, carry out the pricking-cupping bloodletting method on Taiyang, governing vessel, bladder meridian, Quchi, Yanglingquan, Xuehai, Weizhong and the rash, and scrap on Fengchi. It should be noted that the reaction time of the patients with severe pathological steady-state and deep latent disease could be up to a few months. At this time, the mental encouragement and detailed explanation should be given to patients in order to enhance their confidence and understanding.

Appendix

Composition of the Guimen Xiaojie Formula (External use, prohibit internal use):

The equal and moderate amount of Radix Scutellariae, Rhizoma Coptidis, Raw Radix et Rhizoma Rhei, Raw Fructus Gardeniae, Rhizoma Atractylodis, Poria, Raw Radix Glycyrrhizae, Semen Persicae, Radix Paeoniae Rubra and Natrii Sulfas are smashed and soaked in liquor (50% vol) or pure sesame oil for five days.

6. 忽然出现异常咳嗽，以午后和夜间较为明显，部分患者会出现咽喉处梗塞感、上冲感和痛痒感。中医经典《黄帝内经》里曾强调过："一阴一阳结，谓之喉痹。"十二经脉中除手厥阴心包经和足太阳膀胱经外，其余经脉均或直接抵达咽喉，或于咽喉旁经过。至于任脉、冲脉等奇经，也分别循行于咽喉。借助众多经脉的作用，咽喉与全身的脏腑气血发生联系，维持着气机升降出入的正常生理功能。所以通过长期治疗与调理，人体的能量格局一旦发生由否转泰的驱动过程，就会集中反应在这个经脉气血集中而又位置极为特殊的地方。基本处理原则为针刺列缺、照海、丰隆，每日1次，10天为1疗程，常规情况下1疗程内即可明显改善。

7. 绝大多数慢性心脏疾病患者与心脏伴有潜在风险的患者在治疗期间会出现胸闷气短、心慌心悸、乏力疲劳，

6. The patient might have sudden abnormal cough especially after noon and at night. And some patients could have senses of infarction, upflushing, pain and itch in the throat. It has been emphasized in *Huangdi Neijing* that "Stagnation of the pathogenic factors in one Yin and one Yang causes swelling and obstruction of the throat". In the twelve meridians, except the pericardium and bladder meridian, the other meridians either reach the throat directly or pass by the throat. As for some of the extra meridians such as conception vessel and thoroughfare vessel, they also pass through the throat. With the support of a wide range of meridians, the throat is connected with the Qi, blood and Zang-fu organs of the whole body, and the normal physiological functions of ascent, descent, exit and entry of the Qi movement also depend on it. Therefore, through long-term treatment and conditioning, once the energy pattern of the human body is driven, the dizziness reaction will focus on the throat, an extremely special position where the meridians, Qi and blood are concentrated. The basic treatment principle is to take the acupuncture at Lieque, Zhaohai and Fenglong. The patients should be treated 10 days as a course once a day, and the dizziness reaction could be significantly relieved after a course of treatment in general.

7. Most patients with chronic heart disease or potential risk of heart may experience chest stifling oppression, palpitation, fatigue and even different degrees of pain, sense

甚至伴有不同程度的疼痛感、濒死感与烦躁感。（注意与急性心肌梗死相鉴别，此处应介入心电图、血清心肌酶和肌钙蛋白检查，如诊断为急性心肌梗死，务必及时介入西医治疗。）这是治疗期间药势与病势的核心矛盾聚集于厥阴心包附近的焦膜系统，加之病理产物较长时间的积聚，经络淤堵较重，正气来复、逼邪外出时出现了短时间内能量结构凝滞的生理状态。这也进一步提醒我们深入探究癌前病理期与心脏病理期的部分正相关性。中医理论认为，心为君主之官，其余分属脏腑可代君主受邪，故心脏本身癌变的情况在临床中十分罕见，但这却不能屏蔽掉癌变在人体内发生的可能性。基本处理原则为嘱咐患者舌下含服麝香保心丸或口服通心络胶囊，并合用重剂通脉四逆汤，配合适当的吸氧治疗（长期、持续、低流量吸氧）。针刺患者双侧内关，施以小幅度高频率捻转与小幅度提插复式补法1分钟后向对侧外关透刺，针尖不透皮，以皮下可以看到针尖活动为度，尺泽青筋处刺络放血，血变则止，膻中、鸠尾、至阳、胸痛胸闷后背对应放射区予以拔罐，以局部紫红为度，起罐后予以持续按压至阳（俯卧位最佳）、膻中透刺鸠尾并长时间留针，针刺关元并施以呼吸补法，

of impending death and dysphoria during the treatment. (Pay attention to the identification of acute myocardial infarction, and the electrocardiogram, serum myocardial enzymes and troponin should be involved in the examination. If diagnosed as acute myocardial infarction, it is important to introduce modern medicine treatment in time.) This is the core contradiction between the drugs potential and pathogenic factors gathering in the triple energizer membrane system of the heart during the treatment, and together with the long-term accumulation of pathological products and the serious siltation of meridians, the short-term physiological state of stagnant energy structure caused by recovered healthy Qi dispelling the pathogenic Qi is formed. This further reminds us to explore the partial positive correlation between precancerous and heart pathological stage deeply. The TCM theory holds that the heart is the monarch of the body, and the other Zang-fu organs can replace it to be affected by the pathogenic Qi. Therefore, the carcinogenesis of the heart itself is very rare in clinic, while the possibility of the carcinogenesis in other parts of the human body is not low. The basic treatment principles are to take Shexiang Baoxin Pills or Tongxinluo capsule with high dose of Tongmai Sini Decoction combined with appropriate oxygen inhalation therapy (long-term, continuous and low flow oxygen inhalation), take the acupuncture at Neiguan with double-tonification method (Apply small-amplitude and high-

治疗过程中应嘱咐患者同时配合腹式呼吸。每日1次，10天为1疗程，常规情况下1～2疗程内即可明显改善。另由于心脏焦膜系统功能的特殊性与病理稳态的顽固性，多数患者会在一定阶段内反复发作，而非治疗上的一劳永逸，加之反应濒死感带给患者的恐惧，故应提前与患者进行沟通与诱导，关键时刻患者家属与医生也应陪护患者身边，为患者的治疗提供信心与动力。

8. 一定疗程后部分患者会出现头晕目眩、头痛难忍、

frequency twisting and small-amplitude lifting and thrusting for 1 minute) and then join to the opposite Waiguan (The tip of the needle is not transdermal, and the activity of the tip can be seen under the skin), carry out pricking collaterals and bloodletting at the prominent veins of Chize, cup on Tanzhong, Jiuwei, Zhiyang and the corresponding area of chest stifling oppression on the back, press Zhiyang continuously after cupping (Prone position is preferred), take the joining acupuncture from Tanzhong to Jiuwei and retain the needle for a long time, and take the acupuncture at Guanyuan with breathing reinforcement. (Patients should be instructed to cooperate with abdominal breathing at the same time during the treatment.) The patients should be treated 10 days as a course once a day, and the dizziness reaction can be significantly relieved after 1~2 courses of treatment in general. It should be emphasized that because of the function particularity of triple energizer membrane system of the heart and the stubbornness of pathological homeostasis, most of the patients' dizziness reaction will attack repeatedly in a certain stage rather than once and for all in treatment coupled with the possible sense of impending death brought to patients. The advanced communications and inducements with patients are extremely necessary. And during the critical moment, the family members and doctors should also accompany the patients to provide confidence and motivation for the treatment.

8. After a certain course of treatment, some patients

恶心乏力的表现，甚者卧床不起，高血压和低血压的患者都有可能会伴有血压的明显波动。中医理论认为，头为清窍，是人体的诸阳之会。治疗期间气血涌动涤荡重新深度修复人体格局时，可能会重新进入中医认为的原始混沌境界。在此期间，邪气上逆则会引起血压的明显升高而头痛头晕，死阴浮外则会引起血压的明显降低而恶心乏力。由此我们也可以进一步探究，治疗期间血压的波动可能是人体内部正邪相抟、气血涌动的一种外在表现形式，故而患者的癌前病理状态也应与血压有着特殊的病理联系，即癌症的发生过程可能会引起血压的异常波动，而不同的血压异常持续状态也会引起患者呈现出不同的癌变方向性。基本处理原则为针对血压明显异常者，针刺双侧人迎（垂直进针，快速透皮缓慢刺入5分左右，使针尖抵靠触及颈动脉壁，针柄会随动脉同时搏动，留针10分钟）。血压高者配以合谷、太冲（叉刺法），百会放血，呈高血压危象者，可短期内予以西药强化治疗。血压低者配以曲池、足三里，温灸百会。头痛者针刺百会，配以双侧太阳、印堂拔罐，以局部紫红为度，外加双侧风池刮痧（手法从上往下）。恶心乏力者针刺双侧内关，施以小幅度高频率捻转

might have dizziness, intolerable headache, nausea, fatigue and even bedridden condition. Patients with hypertension and hypotension may be accompanied by obvious fluctuations in blood pressure. The TCM theory holds that the head is filled with clear orifices and is the confluence of the Yang meridians. During the treatment, the human body may re-enter the original chaotic realm considered by TCM when the energies of Qi and blood are activated to restore it in depth. During this period, the counterflow ascend of pathogenic Qi will lead to the obvious increase of blood pressure, headache and dizziness, and the emergence of dead-yin will lead to the obvious decrease of blood pressure, nausea and fatigue. From this, we can further explore that the fluctuation of blood pressure during the treatment may be a kind of external manifestation of internal struggle between healthy and pathogenic Qi and activation of Qi and blood energy, so the precancerous pathological state of patients may also have a special pathological connection with the blood pressure. In other words, the occurrence of cancer may cause abnormal fluctuation of the blood pressure, and different abnormal states of blood pressure will also cause different cancerous directions of the patients. The basic treatment principle for the patients with obvious abnormal blood pressure is to take the acupuncture at both sides of Renying (Enter the needle vertically, penetrate the skin quickly and stab slowly into

与小幅度提插复式补法，中脘拔罐。每日1次，10天为1疗程，常规情况下1～2疗程即可明显改善，平素血压异常者疗程相应延长，长者可达数月。治疗期间务必嘱咐患者活动幅度与频率宜轻宜缓，建议卧床休息，不要继续劳作，以防发生意外。另外要注意现代常规ACEI降压制剂的致肺癌隐患，虽然有临床试验结果发现抗高血压治疗与心血管事件的减少有良好的相关性，但目前并没有任何临床试验可以证明降压药能够直接降低患者心血管事件发生的概率，相反，长期服用降压药会加重人体相应部位的缺血、缺氧状态，最终导致机体神经—内分泌—免疫的内环境紊乱，反而会增加心脑血管疾病发生的风险。

the point about 0.5 inches. Make the tip of the needle lean against the wall of the carotid artery, and the handle of the needle will beat with the artery at the same time. Then retain the needle for 10 minutes). Hegu, Taichong (With fork-acupuncture method) and bloodletting on Baihui could be combined with it if the blood pressure is high (Patients with hypertension crisis can be treated with western medicine in a short period of time); Quchi, Zusanli, and moxibustion on Baihui could be combined with it if the blood pressure is low. For the patients with headache, take the acupuncture at Baihui, cup on both sides of Taiyang and Yintang and scrap on both sides of Fengchi (From top to bottom); For the patients with nausea and fatigue, take the acupuncture at Neiguan with double-tonification method (Apply small-amplitude and high-frequency twisting and small-amplitude lifting and thrusting for 1 minute) and cup on Zhongwan. The patients should be treated 10 days as a course once a day, and the dizziness reaction can be significantly relieved after 1~2 courses of treatment in general. The course of treatment of patients with previous hypertension or hypotension may be prolonged up to a few months accordingly. During the treatment, it is extremely necessary to tell the patients that the range and frequency of activity should be light and slow and make them go to bed for rest in time and avoid tiring activities in case of accidents. In addition, attention should be paid to

9. 服药期间出现类似感冒的症状。六经皆有表证，外感是表证中最具典型性的病理雏形，治疗期间机体可多次通过表证的生理反馈与连锁反应而实现人体免疫系统的规律性更新与修复。以发热为例，发热主要是为了提高机体的代谢率，它实际上是 EP 分子在交叉促进与帮助体内免疫系统良性应激过程中的一个附属生命活动，促进免疫应答是其核心目的，一旦出现了在临床治疗中可控、可操作的正邪交争的"调定点"，我们就会有更大的治疗契机与把握。所以，促进人体正气恢复、自我排邪的趋势是中医治疗任何疾病的关键。基本处理原则为立足六经辨证，顺

the potential risk of lung cancer of the modern conventional ACEI blood pressure medication. Although there is a good correlation between the anti-hypertension treatment and the reduction of the cardiovascular events in the clinical trial results, there is no clinical trial can be used to prove that the blood pressure medication is capable of directly reducing the probability of the occurrence of cardiovascular events. On the contrary, taking blood pressure medication for a long time will aggravate the ischemia and hypoxia of the corresponding parts of the human body, which will eventually lead to the disorder of neuroendocrine-immune internal environment, and increase the risk of cardiovascular and cerebrovascular diseases.

9. The patient might have symptoms of similar cold during the treatment. All the six meridians have exterior syndromes, and the common cold is the most typical pathological form in exterior syndromes. During the treatment, the human body can realize the regular update and repair of the immune system through the physiological feedback and the chain reaction of exterior syndrome. Taking the fever as an example, the fever is mainly to improve the metabolic rate of the body, and it is actually an accessory life activity in the process of EP molecule cross-promoting and helping the Eustress of the immune system in the body. Promoting immune response is its core purpose, and once there is a controllable and operable "adjustment point" of

应人体排病之势，随证治之。值得注意的是，大部分类似外感的症状即便在不介入中药的情况下于1～4天内亦可实现自愈。

10. 忽然腹中疼痛或腹内寒热不调，患者矢气泄泻频频，甚者恶心呕吐、不欲饮食或出现身体眼目发黄。这是因为治疗期间正气来复通过逆向主动调节将人体经脉和脏腑内潜伏已久的浊阴之邪通过三焦膜腠代谢化动到消化道而排出（脾胃中土，万物所归）。这本身与消化道消化、吸收的功能与作用方向完全相反，所以人体为了顾全疾病主要矛盾和转归态势，会暂时屏蔽消化吸收的生理过程，专注于给邪以出路，自然也就会出现不欲饮食、恶心呕吐下利的反应，短期内会出现面黄肌瘦（部分患者亦会出现"阴黄"，此类患者大多肝脾运转功能很差，可能有消化系统的癌变隐患），犹如大病一场。在此期间患者容易心生恐惧与挫败感，但要记住，这也是治愈最核心也最为关键的时期。中医理论认为脾胃是人体最核心的枢纽，脾胃中

struggle between healthy Qi and pathogenic Qi in clinical treatment, we will have a greater opportunity and grasp of treatment. Therefore, to promote the recovery of healthy Qi and self-detoxification of the human body is the key to the TCM treatment of any disease. The basic treatment principle is based on the syndrome differentiation of the six meridians. It is worth noting that most patients with cold-like symptoms could recover within 1~4 days even without TCM treatment.

10. The patient might suddenly have abdominal pain, abdominal cold and heat disorders, frequent flatus and diarrhea, and even nausea and vomit, inappetence or jaundice. This is because the restored healthy Qi metabolizes the long-standing pathogenic factors of meridians and Zang-fu organs to the digestive tract for expelling through the triple energizer membrane and reverse active adjustment during the treatment. (The TCM theory holds that the digestive system governs center-earth, and the metabolism of human being is rooted on it.) This metabolic process itself is completely opposite to the function and direction of digestive tract digestion and absorption. So in order to take into account the main contradiction and the outcome of the whole pathological process, the human body itself will temporarily block the physiological process of digestion and absorption and focus on creating conditions for the expulsion of pathogenic factors, and the patients will have symptoms such as inappetence,

气带动四维阴阳升降。而大多数患者在得病时的身体状态都是中国上古经典《周易》里所讲的"否卦"之象。否卦是《易经》六十四卦的第十二卦,天地否,不交不通,则万物不能逐其生,不能通顺和达于四方而万事咽阻。否卦,意预着由安泰到混乱、由通畅到闭塞、由清明到晦暗,黑暗势力增长、正义力量势消的动荡时期,可以认为是一种阴阳否格的状态。通过长时间治疗量变引起质变的过程,"否极泰来"的能量格局在体内的巨变也一定会出现"盘古开天地"的效应,患者也必然会"大死一番",而后"浴火重生"。基本处理原则为针刺合谷(叉刺)、内关、曲池、中脘、天枢、关元、阳陵泉、阴陵泉(沿太阴脾经循行逆方向呈30°进针1.5~2寸)、足三里、上巨虚、下巨虚、丰隆、三阴交(沿胫骨内侧缘呈45°进针1~1.5寸)、太冲(叉刺),施以适当手法,以出现麻电放射感为度,腹部疼痛后背对应放射区予以拔罐,以局部紫红为度。每日1次,10天为1疗程,常规情况下1~2疗程即可明显改善。

nausea, vomit and diarrhea. Some patients will appear to be sallow and emaciated in the short term as if suffering a severe illness. (Some patients with poor function or hidden danger of canceration of the digestive system will also have "Yin jaundice" during the treatment.) During this period, patients are prone to have senses of fear and frustration, but we should keep in mind that this is also the most critical period of cure. The TCM theory holds that the spleen and stomach are the most core hubs of the human body, and the middle Qi of the spleen and stomach drives ascent and descent of Yin and Yang of four different dimensions. The physical state of most patients during this period is the expression of the "Pi Hexagram" of the Chinese ancient classic *Zhouyi*. "Pi Hexagram" is the twelfth hexagram of 64 hexagrams in *Zhouyi*. If there is "Pi" between heaven and earth, it means that the heaven and earth can not interact with each other, which leads to the inability of all living things to conform to their vitality and a state of life energy being blocked. The "Pi Hexagram" indicates a turbulent period from peace to chaos, free to obstruct and clear to dark with the growth of dark forces and the fading of just forces, which can be regarded as a state of stagnation of Yin and Yang. During the long-term treatment of quantitative change leading to qualitative change, the great change of the energy pattern of "Out of the depth of misfortune comes bliss" in the body is bound to have the

11. 2型糖尿病患者的血糖指标可能会升高。现代病理学认为2型糖尿病是诱发癌症的非典型性病理稳态基础。越来越多的证据表明,糖尿病与癌症的关系密切,可增加患癌的风险。后世中医内科学认为糖尿病的病机是本虚标实,临床主要从"火热""阴虚"论治,但大量临床经验表明,这种治疗方式仅仅起到临床初期的缓解作用,绝大多数患者依旧无法摆脱终身服用降糖制剂与并发症的命运。结合癌前病理分析,我们开始逐步意识到2型

effect of "The beginning of the world", and the patients are bound to "die" and "be reborn in the fire". The basic treatment principles are to take the acupuncture at Hegu (With fork-acupuncture method), Neiguan, Quchi, Zhongwan, Tianshu, Guanyuan, Yanglingquan, Yinlingquan (Enter the needle 1.5~2 inches at 30° against the direction of the spleen meridian), Zusanli, Shangjuxu, Xiajuxu, Fenglong, Sanyinjiao (Enter the needle 1~1.5 inches at 45° along the medial edge of the tibia) and Taichong (With fork-acupuncture method) with proper method based on the aim of the occurrence of radiosensitivity, and cup on the corresponding area of bellyache on the back. The patients should be treated 10 days as a course once a day, and the dizziness reaction can be significantly relieved after 1~2 courses of treatment in general.

11. The patients with type 2 diabetes mellitus might have increased indexes of blood glucose. Modern pathology holds that the type 2 diabetes mellitus is an atypical pathological homeostasis basis for inducing cancer. An increasing number of evidences suggest that diabetes is closely related to cancer and can increase the risk of cancer. The later-generation Chinese internal medicine holds that the pathogenesis of diabetes is of deficiency in root and excess in tip and the clinical treatment is mainly based on the "Yin deficiency with effulgent fire", but a great deal of clinical experience shows that this mode of treatment only plays a role in the

糖尿病的本质并非阴虚火旺，实乃李东垣提出的"内伤热中证"的变证，核心病机为脾阳虚衰、气血失运带动人体气机失常、相火不位。治疗期间由于元气蓄积、脾阳复苏，患者则会出现体内气火化动，在此自我修复期间，患者的血糖呈现出与血压波动相类似的表现，但相比血压波动的持续时间，血糖波动的持续时间则会更加漫长，有时会长达 1～2 年不等，对于患者与医生的考验较大。对于绝大多数患者与现代医务人员，血糖持续波动的唯一治疗手段是口服降血糖制剂或胰岛素治疗，而借此维持治疗的患者却无法摆脱部分合并症与癌症的出现，究其本质，是西医学将糖尿病血糖异常表现临床单一化与治疗唯一化的结果。也可以这样理解，血糖异常仅仅是糖尿病的冰山一角，它更像是指示灯，但并不能代表糖尿病发病与治疗的全部。对于 2 型糖尿病根本病因病机的深入探索与发掘，才是颠覆 2 型糖尿病的核心发生过程。基本处理原则为益脾固肾、和解胆枢，在服用中药的同时，可予以温灸大包 30 分钟，针刺阳陵泉、阴陵泉（沿太阴脾经循行逆方向呈 30°进针 1.5～2 寸）、三阴交（沿胫骨内侧缘呈 45°进针 1～1.5 寸）、太溪、太白，施以适当幅度提插手法，

early stage of clinical remission. The vast majority of patients still can't get rid of the fate of life-long hypoglycemic agents and complications. Referring to the precancerous pathological analysis, we have begun to realize gradually that the essence of type 2 diabetes mellitus is not "Yin deficiency with effulgent fire". In fact, it is the "heat-like syndrome of internal damage" put forward by Li Dongyuan. The core pathogenesis of type 2 diabetes mellitus is that the loss of Qi and blood transportation and transformation caused by spleen Yang deficiency leads to the disorder of Qi dynamic and the hyperactivity of ministerial fire. During the treatment, due to the accumulation of the primordial Qi and the recovery of the spleen Yang, the Qi and fire of patients will have a great change in transportation and transformation. And during the self-healing process, the blood glucose fluctuation can appear similar to that of the blood pressure. But compared with the duration of the blood pressure fluctuation, the duration of the blood glucose fluctuation will be longer even for 1 to 2 years, which is a big ordeal for the patients and doctors. For the vast majority of patients and medical staffs, the only targeted measure for continuous fluctuation of blood glucose is oral hypoglycemic preparation or insulin treatment. But the patients who maintain the treatment can not get rid of the emergence of some complications and cancer, that is because the modern clinic deals with the abnormal blood glucose of

以出现麻电放射感为度,每日1次,可呈阶段性持续治疗,以血糖较平稳为度。

12. 二便会出现暂时异常,妇女月经也会出现异于往常的表现。大小便是机体病理产物外排的主要形式,中医理论认为二便与五脏六腑的正常气化功能有着极为密切的联系,故而治疗期间人体脏腑气化功能的调平与恢复会间接引起二便出现异于常态的表现。月经是女性异于男性的独特生理排邪途径,中医理论认为月经与冲脉、任脉、足

diabetes too solely. It can also be understood that abnormal blood glucose is only the "tip of the iceberg" of diabetes. It is more like an "indicator light", but it does not represent the whole process and treatment of diabetes. And it is the core process of overwhelming type 2 diabetes mellitus to explore the fundamental etiology and pathogenesis of type 2 diabetes mellitus. The basic treatment principles are to invigorate spleen and kidney, harmonize gallbladder pivot, take the moxibustion at Dabao for 30 minutes and take the acupuncture at Yanglingquan, Yinlingquan (Enter the needle 1.5~2 inches at 30° against the direction of the spleen meridian), Sanyinjiao (Enter the needle 1~1.5 inches at 45° along the medial edge of the tibia), Taixi and Taibai with proper amplitude lifting-thrusting method based on the aim of the occurrence of radiosensitivity while taking the decoction. The patients should be treated once a day in stages continuously based on the aim of stable blood glucose.

12. The patients might have abnormal stools and urine, and the women's menstruation may be different from usual. The stools and urine are the main forms of the external discharges of the body's pathological products. The TCM theory holds that the stools and urine have a very close connection with the Qi transformation function of the Zang-fu organs, so the harmonization and recovery of the Qi transformation function of the Zang-fu organs can indirectly

阳明胃经、足厥阴肝经、足太阴脾经、足少阴肾经等有着密切的生理与病理联系，故而妇女的月经正常与否直接关系到女性体内气血代谢及正邪盛衰的情况，加之月经期间不停药的基本治疗原则，故而会出现治疗期间月经异于常态的生理性反应，由于其本质归于治疗期间正治与反治的双向调节，故而不作病态看待。基本处理原则为大便秘、排出困难者针刺天枢、足三里、丰隆，每日1次，5天为1疗程，常规情况下1～2疗程即可明显改善。月事疼痛者方中加大芍药用量，外配疼痛后背对应放射区拔罐，以局部紫红为度，同时针刺三阴交（沿胫骨内侧缘呈45°进针1～1.5寸），施以适当幅度提插手法，以出现麻电放射感为度。

cause the stools and urine to become abnormal during the treatment. The menstruation of the woman is a unique physiological detoxification pathway which is different from that of the man. The TCM theory holds that the menstruation has close physiological and pathological relations with thoroughfare channel, conception channel, stomach channel, liver channel, spleen channel, kidney channel, etc. So whether woman's menstruation is normal or not is directly related to the metabolism of Qi and blood and the exuberance and debilitation of the healthy Qi and pathogenic Qi in woman's body. Together with the basic treatment principle of continuous medication during menstruation, there could be abnormal menstrual physiological response during the treatment, and this response should not be treated as morbid state due to its essence boiling down to the two-way regulation of explicable treatment and paradoxical treatment. The basic treatment principle for the patients with constipation is to take the acupuncture at Tianshu, Zusanli and Fenglong 5 days as a course once a day, and the dizziness reaction can be significantly relieved after 1~2 courses of treatment in general. For the patients with dysmenorrhea, the basic treatment principles are to cup on the corresponding area of dysmenorrhea on the back, take the acupuncture at Sanyinjiao (Enter the needle 1~1.5 inches at 45° along the medial edge of the tibia) with proper amplitude lifting-thrusting method based

13. 无精打采，慵懒无力，异常困倦。这是治疗期间阴阳各归其位后身体出现的"休养生息"表现，患者平日的虚性亢奋得以平潜，避免了人体气血不必要的透支与浪费。基本治疗原则为屏蔽掉外界一切干扰，给予身体充分的休息。

14. 对于许多内心世界充满暗能量的患者，治疗期间可能会出现频繁做噩梦的情况，患者梦到的大多是曾经经历过的阴影或是一些比较诡异的事物，有的甚至会出现身心各种原始压力的强烈释放。这就好比阴霾弥漫的冬天遇到了当空烈日，烧灼僭上阴尽，就会出现象征性的"排邪反应"。这期间如果配合适当的心灵疏导，将会起到事半功倍的治疗效果；反之，如果受制于自己的原生阴影而不敢去正视，治疗效果也会大打折扣。我们也发现，在阴影疗愈中患者的立场会不停地将心理动力带到表面，这些大多都是一些原生的恐惧、贪婪或愤怒，治疗会更容易渗入并发挥功效。这两个过程的相互作用发挥的影响，要比

on the aim of the occurrence of radiosensitivity, and increase the dose of Radix Paeoniae Alba in the decoction.

13. The patients might be listless, languid and extremely sleepy. This is the manifestation of rest and recuperation of the body after the Yin and Yang come back to their original position during the treatment. And the ferial deficient Yang with upper manifestation of the patients can be subdued, thus avoiding unnecessary overdraft and waste of Qi and blood in the human body. The basic principles of treatment are to avoid all external interferences and give the body a full rest.

14. The patients with dark energy in the inner world might have frequent nightmares during the treatment. Most of the patients dream of shadows or strange things they have experienced, and some of them may even have a strong release of all kinds of primitive stress of the body and mind. This is like a cloudy winter runs up against the clear sun. The rising and growth of Yang Qi lead to the Yin Qi to be dissipated, and thus there will be a symbolic "exorcism reaction". During this period, the appropriate spiritual guidance can achieve twice the result with half the effort; On the contrary, if the patients are constrained by their own original shadows and dare not to face them squarely, the effect of the treatment will also be greatly reduced. We also find that the patients' positions in the process of shadow healing constantly bring psychological motivation to the surface, most of which are

只运用其一而否定另一种方式带来的效果深刻得多。最终我们得以得出结论：充分暴露矛盾，并将其充分理解与审视，这才是疗愈的根本，而不是一味地逃避与掩盖。而纵观我们中药免疫疗法的癌前介入过程，其核心技术思想也不外乎于此。基本处理原则为结合藏密佛教金刚乘的自他交换法，伴有神经过敏、焦躁多虑而致失眠者同时配合针刺内关（施以小幅度高频率捻转与小幅度提插复式补法1分钟，嘱患者配合腹式呼吸）、四神聪、百会（可长时间留针）。自他交换法是大乘佛教和藏密为了培养众生的解脱慈悲心而创造的独特修行仪轨，这不是一种言论和主观感觉，而是要透过实修让患者的心中真的发展出慈悲心。"自他交换"的练习正是为了斩断那个私我的自我关切、自我助长和自我防卫，让我们逐渐认清我们最恐惧的是：让自己受伤。这个练习不只要我们对别人的苦难产生慈悲心，更要心甘情愿地吸入别人的痛苦，把好的品质吐给他们，这才是真正的大乘慈悲解脱之道。这一点和基督的作为是相同的：承受世人的罪，并因此转化了他们，以及你自己。

native fears, greed or anger, and it makes treatment easier to infiltrate and work. And the interaction between the two processes has a much deeper effect on the treatment than using only one and negating the other. In the end, we can draw the conclusion that it is the root of healing to fully expose the contradiction and fully understand and examine it rather than blindly evading and concealing it. And throughout the precancerous intervention process of TCM immunotherapy, its core technical idea is nothing more than this. The basic principle of treatment is to practise the self-exchange method of Tibetan Vajrayana. For the patients with insomnia caused by susceptibility and anxiety, take the acupuncture at Neiguan (With double-tonification method of applying small-amplitude and high-frequency twisting and small-amplitude lifting and thrusting for 1 minute cooperated with abdominal breathing at the same time), Sishencong and Baihui (The needle can be retained for a long time) at the same time. The self-exchange method is a unique spiritual ritual created by Vajrayana Buddhism in order to cultivate the compassion of all sentient beings. This is not a kind of speech or subjective feeling, but to make the patients' hearts really develop compassion through practical practice. And the self-exchange practice is to cut off the personal self-concern, self-motivation and self-defense, let us gradually realize that what we fear most is to hurt ourselves. This practice requires not only compassion

15. 出现时间规律性发作的病症与反应。中医理论中十二经脉的气血流注都有其特定的对应时间区段，这也决定了治疗期间不同脏腑所属经络可能会出现当令循行所伴随的人体自我修复过程，这也暗含了中药归经理论的部分实存性与规律性。基本处理原则为"病时间时甚者取之输"，即对于时间规律性发作的病理表现可选择发作时间相对应当令循行经络的五输穴中的输穴进行针刺治疗，以病症或反应准备发作前提前针刺为最佳治疗时机。

注：以上所列为瞑眩反应最基本的几种常见情况，因患者的病理基础与病理发展态势不同，临床上亦会伴随出现其他个体特异性反应，基本处理原则可结合六经辨证进行顺势治疗，并充分利用好针灸等外治法的优势，同时要充分权衡中西医诊断与治疗方面的差异性，排除西医病理与诊断对中医治疗的干扰，明晰六经转归至理和中药的特

for the suffering of others, but also willingness to bear the suffering of others and give them good qualities. And it is the real way to extricate ourselves through compassion, which is the same as what Christ did: To bear the sins of the world to transform them and ourselves.

15. The patients might have symptoms and reactions that occur regularly according to the time. The TCM theory is of the opinion that the Qi and blood flows of the twelve meridians have their specific corresponding time zones, which also determines that the meridians belonging to different Zang-fu organs may appear the self-healing process in the corresponding time during the treatment. This also implies the partial solidity and the regularity of the theory of the meridian tropism of Chinese medicines. The basic treatment principle is to take the acupuncture at the transport point of five acupoints of the corresponding meridian of the time zone, and the best treatment time is before the onset of the symptom or reaction.

Note: The symptoms discussed above are the most basic common situations of the dizziness reaction. Because the pathological basis and changes of the patients are different, there will also be other individual specific reactions in clinic. The basic principles of treatment can be based on the six-meridian syndrome differentiation, and we should make full use of the advantages of external treatments such as acupuncture and moxibustion. At the same time, we should

殊属性。

瞑眩反应期间，患者不察、心生胆怯而不配合以及医者胸无定见、治无章法是临证的两大难关，也是临床压力的核心聚焦处。做好医患交流的工作与严密落实临床技术的高水准提升显得尤为重要。结合笔者个人教训，常年积聚在体内的疾病隐患由于被来复之正气所逼，自然无法继续"作祟藏匿"下去，加之疾病"魑魅魍魉"的属性，反而会利用人体正气来复的"瞑眩反应"以动摇患者治疗过程中的正念，甚至会转而采用助长邪气的治疗方式，邪气一旦得到稳固，正气一旦再次遭到打压，患者就会再次深陷之前的病理稳态，甚至身体状况比之前更差。这与恶性肿瘤的经典生物学行为——免疫逃避的作用机制如出一辙。

fully judge and weigh the differences between diagnosis and treatment of traditional Chinese and western medicine, eliminate the interferences of pathology and diagnosis of western medicine to the treatment of TCM, and clarify the dynamic changes of the six meridians and the special properties of TCM.

During the dizziness reaction, there might be patients' incomprehension, fear and noncooperation, and the doctors might treat patients in uncertain opinion or with unorganized method. These are the major clinical difficulties and the core focuses of clinical stress. Therefore, it is particularly important to do good jobs of doctor-patient communication and strictly implement the high level improvement of clinical technology. In the author's opinion, the hidden dangers of the disease which has been accumulating in the body all the year round can not continue to "hide and haunt" because of the restored healthy Qi. But due to the "evil spirit" of the disease, the disease might make use of the dizziness reaction caused by the recovery of the healthy Qi to shake the mindfulness of the patients in the course of treatment, and even lead the patients to switch to the treatment methods that promote the pathogenic Qi. Once the pathogenic Qi is stabilized and the healthy Qi is suppressed again, the patients will once again fall into the pathological homeostasis before, and the physical condition will be even worse than before. This is the same

由此可见，中药免疫疗法的癌前介入对于一个临床医生的心智考验与技术要求极大，加之医患协作方面的复杂性、严谨性与较长时间的临床疗程，注定将成为一个难度极大、跨越性极强的综合性临床医学大型学科。

as the mechanism of immune escape, a kind of classical biological behavior in malignant tumors.

Thus it can be seen that the precancerous intervention of TCM immunotherapy has great mental tests and technical requirements for clinicians. Coupled with the complexity and rigor of doctor-patient cooperation and long periods of clinical treatment, the precancerous intervention of TCM immunotherapy is bound to become a large comprehensive clinical medicine subject with great difficulty and great leapfrogging.

十三、癌前病变的心理社会干预

笔者认为,外在的健康本质上是内在生命力的体现,而许多诸治不愈的疾病背后,大多都会有一个顽固不化的灵魂。同理,个人的生活方式决定健康状态。根据卫生部(现国家卫生健康委员会)相关资料统计,自20世纪90年代后期以来,以慢性病为主生活方式病的死亡人数占总死亡人数的70%以上。恶性肿瘤的新发率与死亡率之高一直是盘踞在21世纪人类生命健康工程之上的挥之不去的巨大阴影,这种"新生物"的骤然突起与凶猛之来势暗合了当今人类社会生活方式的诸多隐患。

诸如食饮五味的极度失衡状态,《黄帝内经》明确指出:"阴之五宫,伤在五味……是故谨和五味,骨正筋柔,气血以流,腠理以密,如是则骨气以精,谨道如法,长有天命。"反观当下社会,烧烤、麻辣烫等"腐败肠胃"之品随处可见,"膏粱厚味"逐渐替代五谷杂粮成为了人们的正餐,水果、冷饮等"闭阻脉门"之物成为了茶余饭后

XIII. Psycho-social Intervention of Precancerous Lesions

The author thinks that the external health is the reflection of inner vitality in essence. And behind many incurable diseases, there may be stubborn souls. Similarly, the personal lifestyle determines the health state. According to the statistics of relevant data of the Ministry of Health (National Health Commission), since the late 1990s, the number of deaths with chronic diseases mainly resulted from unhealthy lifestyle has accounted for more than 70% of the total number of deaths. The high incidence and mortality of malignant tumors have always been lingering shadows over human life and health projects in the 21st century. And the sudden protruding and ferocious emergence of this "new creature" also imply many hidden dangers in the lifestyles in today's human society.

Such as the extremely unbalanced state of the five flavors of diet. The *Huangdi Neijing* has made it clear that "The five Zang-organs that store Yin but also can be damaged by the five flavors...So only when the five flavors are well balanced can the bones be straightened, the sinews be softened, Qi and blood flow smoothly, muscular interstices be intensified and bone Qi be strengthened. Therefore, if we attach importance to the way of diet and implement it in a right way, we will keep

的消遣之品，大量吸烟与酗酒，工作阶层高压力状态下的一日一餐到半夜盛行的夜宵，食品添加剂与地沟油的肆行……这些都明显加重了消化系统肿瘤的发病风险。

笔者在日常生活中也发现，现代人群中绝大部分健身爱好者都会选择夜晚进行运动，殊不知《黄帝内经》有云："阳气者，一日而主外，平旦人气生，日中而阳气隆，日西而阳气已虚，气门乃闭。是故暮而收拒，无扰筋骨，无见雾露，反此三时，形乃困薄"，夜晚肆意挥霍与透支内敛之阳气实为不当之举，长此以往易导致内伤虚劳，即便形体肌肉丰硕，但内在经络脏腑却早已形容枯槁。这也进一步解释了为什么很多人长期健身却又罹患诸多慢性大病，而类似的患者笔者于临证中屡见不鲜。

the vitality of talent for a long time." On the current society, the barbecue, spicy hot pot and other foods that stimulate the intestines and stomach can be found everywhere, the high-fat and high-calorie greasy foods gradually replace the grains and become people's main meals. The foods such as fruits and cold drinks that cause Qi and blood blockade have become recreational snacks after meal. Uncontrolled smoking and drinking, a daily meal under high pressure, midnight snacks, the spread of food additives and gutter oil, etc. significantly increase the risk of digestive system tumors.

In the daily life, the author also finds that the vast majority of fitness enthusiasts will choose to exercise at night, but do not know that "Yang Qi protects the external of the body in the daytime: In the morning, it becomes active; In the noon, it reaches its peak; In the afternoon, it begins to decline and the sweat pores close up accordingly. When it becomes dark, Yang Qi stops moving and stays inside the body, thus the bones and sinews should not be disturbed and care should be taken to avoid being exposed to dew. If one's behavior contradicts the law of these three periods of a day, one's physical appearance will experience distress and weakening" once stressed in *Huangdi Neijing*. It is contrary to the natural law of human body to squander and overdraft the Yang Qi hidden in the body at night. And in the long run, it is easy to lead to internal injury and consumptive disease. Even if the

又如现代人折耗心力、极度焦虑的心理状态,笔者在临证过程中也真切感受到了绝大多数患者低层次与高负压的精神状态。正如 Woody Allen 所说:"我不生气,但我以生肿瘤来替代生气。"从现代流行心理学的观点来看,焦虑消极的情绪会导致疾病的形成。Hagnell 对 2550 名健康人进行了为期 10 年的前瞻性人格研究,发现情绪不稳、易抑郁、不善于表达、转而退缩的人易患肿瘤,他称其为典型的癌前期性格。Temoshok 等提出肿瘤易感性行为特征——"C 型人格",符合这种人格特征的人被形容为外表看上去平静,内心却压抑着许多痛苦的情感;生理上对外界环境的刺激反应强烈,在心理感受上却比较平淡。这种对情绪的压抑、不外泄,有可能通过躯体化的形式表现出来。"最好是成为自由本身,而不只是去瞻仰它,而你的药物不能把你变成自由",这是笔者临证中经常对患者强调的一句话。

bodies and muscles of the patients are strong, the internal meridians and Zang-fu organs have been withered. This further explains why many people work out for a long time but suffer from many chronic serious diseases, and the similar patients are common in the author's clinical experiences.

Another example is the mental state of modern people who are extremely exhausted and anxious, and the author also feels the mental state of the vast majority of patients with low level and high negative pressure during the clinical process. As Woody Allen said: "I'm not angry, but I can replace anger with a tumor." From the point of view of modern pop psychology, negative emotions can lead to diseases. Hagnell, who conducted a 10-year prospective personality study of 2550 healthy people, found that people who were emotionally unstable, depressed, unexpressive and flinching were prone to tumors, and he called it the typical precancerous personality. Temoshok has put forward the behavioral characteristics of cancer-prone — "C-type personality". People who fit this personality are described as one looks calm on the outside, but suppresses a lot of painful feelings in the heart. The stimulation response of this kind of person to the external environment is strong in physiological feeling, but relatively dull in psychological feeling. This kind of suppression of emotion may be manifested in the form of somatization. "It's better to be freedom itself, not just to look to it, and your

由于癌前病变本身是一种慢性病理代偿期，此种病理稳态的形成与患者自身的生活方式有着极为密切的联系。患者经过免疫疗法的系统治疗后，身体虽回复"阴平阳秘"的理想状态，但并非肿瘤防治结果上的一劳永逸。在后期康复与随访过程中，医生务必要落实并完善好相关医嘱和宣教体系，患者务必要彻底改变之前的长期不良生活方式与习惯，有关部门也应做好肿瘤防治的心理社会干预工作与健康科普工作，如此恶性肿瘤的中医药防治网络与防治能力方能实现根本突破。

medicine can't turn yourself into freedom", which the author often emphasizes to the patients in clinic.

Because the precancerous lesion itself is a chronic pathological compensation stage, the formation of this pathological homeostasis is closely related to the patients' own lifestyles. After systematic treatment of immunotherapy, the bodies of the patients return to the ideal state of "relative equilibrium of yin-yang", but it is not once and for all in the result of tumor prevention and treatment. In the process of later rehabilitation and follow-up, the doctors must implement and improve the relevant medical orders and propaganda system, and the patients must completely change the long-term bad lifestyles and habits before, the relevant departments should also do good jobs of psycho-social intervention and health science popularization of tumor prevention and treatment, thus the TCM prevention and treatment network and ability of malignant tumors can achieve a fundamental breakthrough.

十四、结语

纵观全书,我们尝试了以中医经典《伤寒论》为临床启发与切入点,并结合六经整体权变思想、《黄帝内经》反治法、后世各家学派与西医学病生理有关内容,从中发掘癌前病变的病能驱力与本质规律,从而钤以"温补太阴、托透少阴、清宣少阳"的核心基本治法,并按照体质与症候群分类的方法将临证分期、分型、转归及基本处理方式述以大概,将最核心、系统的临证单元与相关技术支持全面呈现给读者。整套方案避免了现代中医临证流于玄化、模糊、泥古、俗套之嫌,将钱学森"现代医学中医化"发挥得淋漓尽致,以全观的学术视野和笃实的学术责任感铸就了理想的临床高度。笔者坚信,随着整套方案与临床科研的推进,中医药的独特优势与魅力将不仅会带给肿瘤学界一股飒爽清风,更会以其大道至简而又不可思议的哲学思维与实证价值感动整个世界。

XIV. Conclusion

Throughout the outline, we have tried to take *Shanghan Lun* as the clinical inspiration and breakthrough point. And referring to the thought of six-meridian syndrome differentiation, the paradoxical treatment method of *Huangdi Neijing*, and the related contents of the TCM later generations' theory and modern pathophysiology, we have found out the driving force and essential rule of precancerous lesions. Thus we are able to refine the core basic treatment method of "warming and supplementing Taiyin, drawing and expelling through Shaoyin, and clearing in Shaoyang". According to the classification of constitution and syndrome, the clinical stage, syndrome differentiation, variation, and basic treatment are presented to the reader in a general way, and the core systematic clinical unit and related technical support are presented comprehensively. The whole scheme rectifies and avoids the suspicion that the clinical flow of TCM is metaphysical, vague, stodgy and threadbare, and gives full play to Qian Xuesen's opinion of "modern medicine in a TCM way". And the ideal clinical height is formed with a comprehensive academic vision and a solid academic sense of responsibility. The author firmly believes that with

最后，笔者欲借唐朝李贺所作《雁门太守行》中"黑云压城城欲摧，甲光向日金鳞开"与宋代陆游所作《游山西村》中"山重水复疑无路，柳暗花明又一村"二句经典诗词与中医临床人共勉，生命临床医学极为复杂而又艰深，而随之伴随的苦涩虚乏之感亦为医学工作者们所皆知，也正是在这种未知黑夜中，我们才得以燃生对光明的渴望，由此祖先的宝贵智慧千年来一直幽微泛烁的火花成为了我们中医人照亮全世界的自信源泉。

the promotion of the whole scheme and clinical scientific research, the unique advantages and charm of TCM will not only bring a cool breeze to the oncology field, but also move the whole world with its simple and incredible philosophical thinking and practical value.

In the end, the author would like to quote from "Dark clouds bearing down on the city threaten to overwhelm it, the light of armour spreads to the sun" written by Li He in the Tang Dynasty and "Where hills bend, streams wind and the pathway seems to end, past dark willows and flowers in bloom lies another village" written by Lu You in the Song Dynasty in the hope of mutual encouragement with TCM clinicians. The clinical medicine of life is extremely complex and difficult, and the accompanying suffering and the sense of deficiency are also known by the medical workers. And it is in this unknown night that we are able to make the desire for light. Thus, the precious wisdom of our ancestors that has been shining sparks for thousands of years has also become the source of confidence for our TCM clinicians to illuminate the world.

参考文献

1. 程书钧. 癌前病变和癌前疾病. 郑州：河南科学技术出版社，2017.

2. 娄绍昆.《内经》反治法新探. 南京中医药大学学报，1991（3）：135-137.

3. 吕英. 气一元论与中医临床. 太原：山西科学技术出版社，2012.

4. Chen Lili,He Zhengxiang,Qin Li,et al.Antitumor Effect of Malaria Parasite Infection in a Murine Lewis Lung Cancer Model through Induction of Innate and Adaptive Immunity. PloS one,2011,6(9),e24407.

5. 陈立华，关茂会，刘燕玲，等. 通阳助阳法治疗乙型肝炎初探. 中医杂志，1986，27（1）27.

6. Benias Petros C,Wells Rebecca G,Sackey-Aboagye Bridget,et al.Author Correction: Structure and distribution of an unrecognized interstitium in human tissues.Scientific reports,2018,8(1),7610.

7. Cronin-Fenton Deirdre.Angiotensin converting enzyme inhibitors and lung cancer.BMJ (Clinical research ed.),2018,363,k4337.

8. 马跃荣,苏宁.病理学.北京:人民卫生出版社,2016.

9. 王冠军,赫捷.肿瘤学概论.北京:人民卫生出版社,2013.

10. 张耕铭.伤寒耕读录 壹:理法方药,医海去芜存菁.北京:中国中医药出版社,2020.

11. 张耕铭.伤寒耕读录 贰:性命双修,医路霹雳精诚.北京:中国中医药出版社,2020.

桶底脱时大地阔,

命根断处碧潭清。

好像一点红炉雪,

散作人间照夜灯。

——［宋］大慧宗杲禅师

The ground suddenly looks vast when the bottom of the bucket falls off,

the inner world tends to be clear when the root of samsara is cut off.

Sprinkle the snow in the fiery stove to the world,

making it a beacon showing the direction in the dark.

— Shi Zonggao, Zen master in Song dynasty